The Cognitive Neuropsychiatry of Parkinson's Disease

The Cognitive Neuropsychiatry of Parkinson's Disease

Patrick McNamara

The MIT Press
Cambridge, Massachusetts
London, England

For information about special quantity discounts, please email special_sales@mitpress.mit.edu

This book was set in Syntax and Times New Roman by Toppan Best-set Premedia Limited. Printed and bound in the United States of America.

Library of Congress Cataloging-in-Publication Data

McNamara, Patrick, 1956–
The cognitive neuropsychiatry of Parkinson's disease / Patrick McNamara.
  p. ; cm.
Includes bibliographical references and index.
ISBN 978-0-262-01608-7 (hardcover : alk. paper)
1. Parkinson's disease. 2. Neuropsychiatry. 3. Cognition. I. Title.
[DNLM: 1. Parkinson Disease—psychology. 2. Cognition—physiology. 3. Mental Disorders—etiology. WL 359]
RC382.M446   2011
616.8′33—dc22

                                                                    2010054271

10   9   8   7   6   5   4   3   2   1

To
Raymon Durso, M.D.
and
Ina Livia McNamara

Contents

Preface   ix
Acknowledgments   xi

1   On Parkinson's Disease   1

2   Dopamine and Parkinson's Disease Neuropsychiatry   25

3   The Nature and Functions of the Agentic Self   37

4   The Neurology of the Agentic Self   57

5   Impairment of the Agentic Self in Parkinson's Disease: Cognitive Deficits in Parkinson's Disease   69

6   The Agentic Self and Personality Changes in Parkinson's Disease   87

7   Evolutionary Perspectives on the Agentic Self, Its Neural Networks, and Parkinson's Disease   111

8   Speech and Language Deficits of Parkinson's Disease   123

9   Sleep Disorders of Parkinson's Disease   137

10   Mood Disorders and Apathy in Parkinson's Disease   155

11   Psychosis and Dementia in Parkinson's Disease   171

12   Impulse Control Disorders in Parkinson's Disease   181

13   Rehabilitation of the Agentic Self   187

References   195
Index   225

Preface

Neuropsychiatric disturbances of Parkinson's disease (PD) can be as disabling as the motor symptoms of the disease, yet these neuropsychiatric disturbances are only recently being intensively studied by clinicians and scientists. Upwards of 85% of PD patients evidence deficits in executive cognitive functions even early in the disease. Almost half of all patients progress toward a dementing illness that may occur late in the disease. More than half of all patients suffer severe anxiety or depression. Roughly 50% of patients suffer varying degrees and types of apathy, hallucinations, sleep disturbance, and impulse control disorders. Despite the devastation these disorders cause the patients and their families, the disorders have not yet received the attention they deserve from the biomedical sciences. Thus, there are few attempts to model theoretically or account for these disorders of PD.

This project describes a new "top-down" approach to neuropsychiatric disorders associated with PD. This is a technical and theoretical work that I hope will, nevertheless, eventually contribute to the development of new treatments for the various afflictions that affect persons with PD and their families. My main goal in this work, however, is not to describe new treatment options for people with PD but to arrive at a better understanding of the human mind and its breakdown patterns in patients with PD.

Traditionally, scientists take a bottom-up approach to the study of any system, object, or phenomena, and this approach, of course, is entirely justified. Examining the simplest possible elements or constituents in or of a system can lead to breakthroughs in identifying ultimate organizing principles, forces, or laws that govern the larger system. However, the top-down approach is worthwhile as well because it, too, can lead to identification of important principles, laws, and elements that govern operation of the larger system. Nowhere is this more clearly the case than in the study of individual human beings or persons. Each individual or person is utterly unique in myriad ways (memory content, behavioral preferences and desires, belief systems, knowledge base, and so on). To some extent then (and one must *not* take this claim too far), one (not the primary but one) purpose of the human mind/ brain is to build a person. The whole physiologic apparatus is to some extent designed to create this self structure or person. The human mind/brain can be seen as an elaborate, complex, and grotesquely baroque construction or "Rube Goldberg machine" patched together to produce this fragile thing we call the self. When the self structure is disrupted in a particular way, you get the breakdown patterns we see in various neuropsychiatric disorders, including the disorders we see in PD. By observing its breakdown patterns in PD, we get a glimpse into the inner workings of that most spectacular of structures of the self system—the agentic self, the self that acts. That at least is what I hope to demonstrate in this monograph.

Acknowledgments

I would like to thank Robert Prior from the MIT Press for supporting this project. I would like to extend a special thanks to Ms. Erica Harris, my head research coordinator, who helped out on all aspects of this book project. In addition, I would like to thank Erica for her extensive comments on an earlier draft of this book and for her work on apathy in persons with PD, which I drew from for this monograph. I thank Prof. Thomas Holtgraves for teaching me the basics of the idea of language as social action. Most of our experiments reported in the chapter on speech and language deficits of PD (chapter 8) were designed by him.

I thank also the thousands of individuals with PD that I have had the privilege of meeting and working with over the years. Their courage and their good humor in trying circumstances have been an inspiration for me.

This work was supported, in part, by the Office of Research and Development, Medical Research Service, Department of Veterans Affairs and by NIDCD grant no. 5R01DC007956–03.

This book is dedicated to Dr. Raymon Durso, a longtime collaborator, colleague, and mentor. He, more than anyone else, has instructed me in the intricacies and complexities of PD—most especially, he has insisted that I not lose sight of the humanity of these individuals, that I not forget that these are people and families trying to cope with an impossible and relentless disease, and that what defines them are their strengths, not their deficits. They are not just "patients" but are instead "agents" striving to realize what is best for themselves, their families and their communities. That is why I focus on the agentic self in PD in this book.

1 On Parkinson's Disease

This book presents a theory concerning certain symptoms associated with the major neuropsychiatric disorders of Parkinson's disease (PD). We will, therefore, need to present the basics of PD for readers not familiar with the condition.

PD is a progressive neurodegenerative disorder that most commonly strikes people over 60 years of age. The mean duration of the disease is approximately 13 years, and the mean age at death is approximately 73. Its cardinal clinical manifestations are four major motor deficits: resting tremor, rigidity, bradykinesia, and gait dysfunction. I will discuss these fundamental motor problems more thoroughly later. PD, however, is also associated with many nonmotor deficits, including autonomic dysfunction, pain, mood disorders, sleep problems, and cognitive impairment. Both the motor and the nonmotor deficits of PD are due, in part, to degeneration of pigmented dopaminergic neurons in the substantia nigra pars compacta (SNc) coupled with intracytoplasmic proteinaceous inclusions known as Lewy bodies. There is degeneration in all of the other major neurotransmitter nuclei (e.g., the noradrenergic locus caeruleus, the serotonergic raphe nucleus, etc.) as well, but given that the motor deficits and some of the nonmotor deficits of PD can be partially reversed or alleviated by dopamine replacement therapy, it is reasonable to assume that loss of midbrain dopamine contributes significantly (but not solely) to these motor and some of the nonmotor (neuropsychiatric/cognitive) deficits of PD.

This book is concerned primarily with the neuropsychiatric and cognitive deficits of PD, though I believe the nonmotor features of PD are significantly influenced by the motor dysfunction of the disease. Both the motor and nonmotor features of the disease are partially due to and shaped by reduction in the magnitude of phasic bursting in dopaminergic terminals that carry predicted error signals vis-à-vis motor outputs and behavioral actions. I will be arguing that the cognitive, mood, and personality changes of PD are essentially due to inability to activate fully agentic aspects of the self that (as I will show in a later chapter) are themselves rooted in motor and cognitive control system dynamics that depend on phasic bursting in nigrostriatal, basal ganglia, and mesocortical dopamine systems.

What Is Parkinson's Disease?

Parkinson's disease is the second most common neurodegenerative disorder (after Alzheimer's disease) with an estimated 5 million affected people throughout the world. These numbers should rise as populations age and environmental toxins proliferate (age and toxins are two major risk factors for PD).

Men are twice as likely as women to develop PD. Estrogens may offer some protection against PD, as when women develop PD, they develop it at an older age on average than do men. If men have the disease, they manifest motor symptoms of PD at about age 60, but if women have PD, they typically manifest the motor symptoms at age 62 or 63. In the first few years of the disease, women, on average, also exhibit less severe motor deficits but more severe treatment-related dyskinesias. Dyskinesias are uncontrollable and sometimes painful jerky and jumpy movements and motor tics.

A notable recent study (Gao, Simon, Han, Schwarzschild, & Ascherio, 2009) suggested that people with red hair had an approximately twofold higher risk for PD relative to those with black hair. People who carried a gene mutation that influences both skin and hair color (MC1R Arg151Cys variant allele) had a significantly increased risk for PD. This gene presumably influences levels of melanin and neuromelanin in the person's body. Independent studies of the cell loss in PD have demonstrated that severity of PD is associated with loss of pigment-containing cells of the substantia nigra—the cells that produce dopamine. If people with red hair have lower baseline levels of these pigmented cells in the substantia nigra, then they would be more vulnerable to PD if and when it strikes. There is also an older body of literature (reviewed in Geschwind & Galaburda, 1985a–c, 1987) that suggests that hypopigmented individuals (like people with red or blond hair) also tend to be less strongly right-handed than other people. Non-right-handedness, in turn, sometimes indexes less lateralization in brain organization. For example, people with various neuropsychiatric disorders exhibit less strongly lateralized ear preferences and hand preferences. If that is indeed the case, then hypopigmented people with PD may be at greater risk for certain types of neuropsychiatric disorder compared with that of non-hypopigmented people with PD because of the reduced asymmetry that characterizes the brains of hypopigmented individuals. But all of this is as yet speculation. We will see below that there are other less "colorful" reasons (besides reduced asymmetry) to expect neuropsychiatric disorders in PD.

History of Study of PD

Although PD was likely known to the ancients, it was not seriously studied until the medieval period (apparently by the Islamic philosopher Averroes). PD was not well recognized in the ancient world probably because not many people lived into their sixties or seventies in that time, so PD must have been more rare in the ancient world than it is today. The scientific study of PD did not commence until James Parkinson published his "Essay on the shaking palsy" in 1817 when he was 62. Parkinson based his analyses on clinical observations of six patients, three of them "from a distance." Apparently, he observed and talked with these three only on the street and not in his clinic. Despite this paucity of material, he managed to identify the major motor deficits and postural abnormalities of the disease. Whereas he recognized delirium as one possible outcome of the progression of the disease, he did not seem to think that intellectual or cognitive deficits were part of the intrinsic nature of the disease. As physicians became more aware of Parkinson's monograph, "paralysis agitans" began to be recognized as a clinical syndrome in its own right.

Jean-Martin Charcot (1825–1893) was a celebrated French neurologist working at the Salpêtrière Hospital in Paris. He knew about Parkinson's monograph but had trouble getting a copy of it. He had been making systematic observations of patients with paralysis agitans (though Charcot did not like that name for the disease) for years. Once he got a copy of Parkinson's essay, Charcot added new symptoms that characterized the disease in terms similar to those described by Parkinson. He suggested that the disease be named after Parkinson, and from that point on, the signs and symptoms of PD were recognized as a syndrome, or collection of symptoms, that likely had a common cause. Charcot did not stop at clinical observation of the disease. He also devised all kinds of therapies to treat the disease including an innovative vibration therapy. He had noticed that some PD patients felt better after they had undergone bone-jarring carriage or train rides. He developed an automated vibratory chair (fauteuil trépidant; Goetz, 2009) and had patients sit in it for 30-minute sessions and then observed improvement in symptoms. Oddly enough, this innovative therapeutic strategy was never followed up after Georges Gilles de la Tourette developed a helmet that vibrated the head on the premise that the brain was the crucial site of action for the disease. Whereas Gilles de la Tourette was correct in that assumption, he was incorrect in assuming that vibrating the head would necessarily yield greater therapeutic benefit. When the vibratory helmet seemed unimpressive in its effects, new therapeutic innovation to treat PD slowed considerably.

In the early decades of the twentieth century, a flu epidemic swept the world. Some victims of this epidemic developed signs of PD and their cases were studied intensively, thus advancing knowledge of the parkinsonian symptoms. Neuropathologic studies of the brainstems of some of these patients yielded clues as to brain lesions that might cause PD symptoms. In the 1950s, the most crucial discovery in PD science was made when the substantia nigra, a site associated with the production of dopamine, was identified as a site of damage in parkinsonian syndromes. In 1960, dopamine was found to be decreased in the brains of people with PD. In 1961–1962, the first successful trials of levodopa occurred. Levodopa is an amino acid precursor to the biochemical synthesis pathway that manufactures dopamine. By increasing dopamine's precursor, the chances that more dopamine would be manufactured in the brain itself increased. By 1968, patients were being treated with levodopa and with spectacular success.

Levodopa (L-dopa; LD) therapy worked so well for some patients that it seemed that they could live relatively normal lives. This was the dramatic breakthrough everyone had been hoping for. Could people be cured simply by taking a supplement? It was soon discovered, however, that LD had unpleasant side effects (nausea and dyskinesias) and could not prevent progression of the disease. Attention turned to finding ways to ameliorate the unpleasant side effects of LD. The nausea was soon brought under control by the addition of a peripheral dopamine blocker. LD increased both central and peripheral dopamine, and when it did so in the periphery, it created severe nausea. However, a drug called carbidopa could block the synthesis of dopamine in the periphery, and when added to LD, the new drug combination worked pretty well. Nevertheless, no solution has yet been found for the dyskinesias that plague many patients on LD, nor has it been possible to slow progression of the disease.

In an effort to augment LD or to ameliorate some of its dyskinetic side effects, new catecholaminergic drugs like bromocriptine and the monoamine oxidase (MAO)-B inhibitor deprenyl were developed in the 1970s. Pergolide, selegiline, and antioxidant therapies were developed in the 1980s. Meanwhile, deep brain stimulation therapies were introduced in the late 1980s, and neurosurgical techniques were refined in the 1980s and 1990s. In 1997, the U.S. Food and Drug Administration (FDA) approved use of deep brain stimulation (DBS) of the subthalamic nucleus for treatment of tremor. By stimulating the subthalamic nucleus, one could release from inhibition targets downstream from the nucleus that controlled motor output and thus improve some motor functions in PD. Throughout the 1990s, many of the genetic defects that have been implicated in PD were discovered. Identification of these genetic abnormalities and their associated metabolic effects would lead to new therapies that targeted those metabolic defects in the 2000s. A gene therapy (that did not work so well) for PD was introduced in 2005. Gene therapies, neuroprotective therapies, antiapoptotic therapies, complementary and alternative medicine (CAM) therapies, and all kinds of other therapies as well have been developed in the first decade of the twenty-first century. None of these therapies, however, have yet proved able to prevent progression of the disease or the dyskinesias, though DBS seems to help some people sometimes with dyskinesias and other PD symptoms.

In a recent study (Weaver et al., 2009) of more than 200 advanced-stage PD patients, researchers found that DBS was more effective than standard forms of therapy in improving drug "on time" (when good motor response to LD was achieved). Patients in the DBS group gained as much as 4½ hours of on time compared with that of the control therapy group. In DBS, electrodes are implanted in the brain and connected to a small electrical device called a pulse generator that can be controlled by the patient and/or the doctor. DBS is used to stimulate those brain regions that have been damaged by the disease. The study involved patients with bilateral implantation of stimulators, meaning that devices were implanted on both sides of the brain. Unilateral forms of implantation carry fewer risks, but of course DBS of any kind requires surgery, and surgery always carries significant risks when compared to less invasive therapies.

The Gold Standard Therapy for PD and Its Vicissitudes

The gold standard treatment for PD is LD. In the first couple of years of the disease, LD practically normalizes the motor deficits of PD for most, but not all, patients with PD. Unfortunately, it does this for only a certain amount of time and over only a certain number of years. The side effects of LD such as nausea, dyskinesia, and low blood pressure have been minimized by the creation of Sinemet, which is a combination of carbidopa and LD. Carbidopa is a dopa decarboxylase inhibitor that potentiates the effect of LD by modifying the body's metabolism of the substance so that it is not converted to dopamine until it reaches the brain. In most countries, carbidopa/LD dose levels are designated as a fraction. For example, a 25/100 prescription indicates that the pill is composed of 25 mg carbidopa and 100 mg LD.

To augment use of dopamine in the brain and potentially reduce the side effects of LD (like dyskinesias), other dopaminergic agents besides LD have been developed. The agonists act directly on dopamine receptors, whereas the catechol-*O*-methyltransferase (COMT) and MAO inhibitors act to inhibit breakdown of existing depots of dopamine in the system. There are several types of dopamine agonists: bromocriptine (Parlodel), pergolide (Permax), pramipexole (Mirapex), ropinirole (Requip), lisuride, and cabergoline. All of these agonists are important in the story of impulsivity syndromes in PD, so we will have occasion to speak of them again in that chapter. These agonists stimulate dopaminergic activity in the reward centers of the brain by stimulating D_2 receptors. Pramipexole and ropinirole in addition stimulate D_3 receptors. Because the D_3 receptor is involved in mood, personality, and emotion, pramipexole and ropinirole may affect mood as well as motor symptoms. All of these agonist drugs also affect cognitive functions, usually working memory functions, as well. The COMT inhibitors, such as tolcapone (Tasmar) and entacapone (Comtan), act to use existing dopamine levels (by inhibiting the breakdown of dopamine by COMT in the synaptic cleft). The MAO-B inhibitors, such as selegiline (Eldepryl) and rasagiline (Azilect), act to inhibit enzymatic MAO-B activity, which normally breaks down dopamine. Amantadine appears to enhance the activity of both catecholamines (dopamine and norepinephrine). Anticholinergic drugs are sometimes used to decrease cholinergic effects in the motor system that appear to potentiate dyskinesias and other motor problems. See table 1.1 for a list of drugs used to treat PD.

The positive effects of dopaminergic therapy for PD are undeniable. People with PD are able to lead largely normal lives for several years after they are diagnosed with the disease. LD therapy also appears to increase life expectancy and may even slow the progression of the disease, though this latter claim is hotly disputed. PD patients treated with LD spend 3 to 5 years more in each Hoehn–Yahr stage compared with patients in the pre-LD era, but it is not yet entirely clear if

Table 1.1
Primary drugs used to relieve the motor symptoms of PD

LD
LD plus peripheral dopa decarboxylase inhibitors (DDIs)
Dopamine receptor agonists
LD plus COMT inhibitors
MAO inhibitors
Anticholinergics
Amantadine

this is due to LD per se or just to better medical treatment more generally. Sporadic neuroimaging findings also suggest that LD may be somewhat toxic to cells that normally manufacture dopamine. However, the jury is still out on this important issue.

Regardless of the outcome of the issue of the effect of LD on dopamine cells, it is clear that LD is associated with the eventual production of disabling motor problems called dyskinesias and motor fluctuations. Duration of exposure to LD, LD dose, PD severity, and age of patient are all strong predictors of dyskinesias and motor fluctuations. Between 50% and 100% of all PD patients taking LD for more than 6 years will develop disabling peak-dose dyskinesias. Various solutions have been offered to handle the problem of dyskinesias and motor fluctuations in PD. These include early use of agonists instead of LD, controlled instead of bolus release of LD, and DBS therapies. All of these techniques have helped but not yet solved the problem of severe motor side effects of LD.

The above are the basic facts of the clinical presentation of PD treatment that the reader will need to know to appreciate the discussion that follows in other chapters on the neuropsychiatric disorders of PD. I will next provide a more in-depth discussion of the natural history of PD symptoms focusing on when and what kind of neuropsychiatric disorders appear at which stage of the disease. Before summarizing the natural history of the disease and its fundamental causes, however, I think it will be valuable to present a few case studies of patients with PD so that the reader can get a feel for the human effects of this disease. I will focus on what the disease does to the self of the patient, but note that each case of PD is unique. There are no hard and fast rules for the effects of PD on the self. Some patients succumb to depression, whereas others wear themselves out with rage against the disease. Most find some balance of acceptance of the limitations that the disease imposes on the self while not allowing the disease to define who they are and what they can do. It is ultimately impossible to capture PD's protean effects on mind and body in any book or summary. Nor is it possible, finally, to capture the courage, good humor, and extraordinary grace that people with PD display when they are confronted with such a devastating disease.

Case Studies

First, I wish to make some general observations on the persistent claim, idea, or "story" that one hears in neurology clinics around the world that a disproportionate number of persons with PD are exceptionally intelligent, ambitious, persistent, meticulous, and dedicated to "their" work (Horowski, Horowski, Calne, & Balne, 2000; Jones, 2004). I personally agree with this story, though I have no data to support it. Nevertheless, my impression is that the kinds of people who develop PD tend to be unusually intelligent and very interested in accomplishment. They tend to be the kind of people who are driven by a desire to achieve something significant, or so the claim goes. Take, for example, the case of Thomas Hobbes (1588–1679), who is best known for his political philosophy, although during his day he was more widely known as a scientist, mathematician, a translator of the Greek classics (such as Thucydides' *Histories*), and as a fierce and passionate writer on religious questions. He developed the "shaking palsy" sometime in the mid-1640s when he was around age 50. He would dictate his works to his secretaries because he could no longer write himself. He wrote the *De Cive* [*On the Citizen*] (1642) right before the onset of his PD, and he wrote his most famous book, *Leviathan*, in 1650–1651, right after onset of the disease. PD, apparently, does not prevent creative work of a very high intellectual caliber, and in some mysterious way (given the timing of Hobbes' greatest works), it may actually promote great creative works—at least in those capable of such great works.

My own subjective impression of the many hundreds of patients with PD that I have worked with over the years agrees with this story concerning people with PD. I will say more about the so-called premorbid personality type of PD in another chapter, but suffice it to say here that among the many unresolved issues concerning those two great disorders that affect midbrain dopaminergic systems, PD and schizophrenia, is the issue of their association with exceptional talent and intelligence in either the patients themselves or their first-degree relatives. The data to support these associations are strong with respect to schizophrenia and still only impressionistic in the case of PD, but I believe those data will eventually support the association of PD and exceptional talent. Nevertheless, I as of yet know of no studies that have compared the percentages of eminent individuals with PD (and their first-degree relatives) with the percentages of eminent persons with a similar long-term neurologic illness like multiple sclerosis or Huntington's disease or even schizophrenia. See box 1.1 for names of some famous people who are known or suspected to have had PD.

I now turn to some recent cases of PD. It may be instructive to begin with two cases of prominent people with PD and then turn to two cases of nonfamous but arguably equally intelligent and accomplished people with PD.

Pope John Paul II had been something of an athlete in his youth. He particularly loved to hike in the mountains and to ski. After becoming a priest, he rose rapidly

Box 1.1
Famous People Suspected of Having PD

Here are some famous politicians, good and bad, who either are known to have had PD or are strongly suspected to have had PD:

Senator Claiborne Pell of Rhode Island (1918–2009)

Governor George Wallace of Alabama (1919–1998)

Mayor John Lindsay of New York (1921–2000)

Prime Minister Enoch Powell of Britain (1912–1998)

Prime Minister Pierre Trudeau of Canada (1919–2000)

Chairman Mao Zedong of China (1893–1976)

Deng Xio Ping of China (successor to Mao) (1904–1997)

Francisco Franco of Spain (1892–1975)

in the ranks of the Roman Catholic hierarchy, very ably representing his Polish flock as bishop during the years of communist rule in Poland. After becoming pope, he faced one crisis after another with aplomb and intelligence. He served as pope for 12 years after receiving the diagnosis at age 72. As with most other persons with PD, the disease itself probably began some years before the diagnosis. If so, that would indicate that for the majority of his pontificate (that lasted some 25 years), he had suffered from some degree of PD. He is credited by most historians with playing a crucial role in the peaceful overthrow of the Polish communist dictatorship during the late 1980s. He wrote thousands of pages of religious texts as well as plays and philosophical treatises. His papal encyclicals were considered masterpieces by many. He even had a few bestsellers on the spirituals lists! He had survived an assassination attempt in 1981, and throughout his pontificate, he kept up a physical pace that made the young people around him breathless. He traveled virtually every year, ultimately visiting some 129 countries outside of Italy itself. After he developed PD, he regularly called attention to the disease during his papal audiences and met several times with representatives of PD service organizations, hoping to boost their efforts at serving the PD community. Taken together, this man's accomplishments, despite the PD, have to be reckoned impressive and even extraordinary. Perhaps the Vatican obscured any neuropsychiatric disorders that the pope grappled with due to his PD, but if so, it would constitute a miracle of media management tactics as the man was constantly in the public eye right up to his death. Did he grapple with depression, apathy, anxiety, or even sleep problems (all common disorders associated with PD)? We do not know. He clearly evidenced speech and language problems in the last years of his life. We will cover speech and language disorders of PD in another chapter, but that is about all we know of the pope's PD, besides the crucial fact that the man flourished despite the PD.

The actor Michael J. Fox was diagnosed with PD at the very young age of 29. Thus, he has lived with the disease for well nigh 20 years. Instead of retiring from the world after he received the diagnosis, he created a charitable foundation that has raised an enormous amount of money to fund PD research, especially research that focuses on the creation of immediate ameliorative therapies for patients and their families. The Michael J. Fox Foundation has taken a leadership role in the PD advocacy community and thus has immeasurably enriched the lives of all PD patients and their families. Like Pope John Paul II, Michael J. Fox travels the world doing dozens of interviews, meeting with politicians of every stripe and variety, conducting nonstop fundraisers, asking for money from the rich and powerful, and, unlike the former pope, doing all this while raising a family of four kids! Although PD must have slowed him down in some crucial respects, it is hard to see how. In his memoirs, Fox displays a healthy sense of humor about his PD symptoms, describing scene after scene of his dyskinesias intruding into meetings with the rich and famous. Fox says that he has never struggled with depression, but he also understands that he has been unusually lucky in this regard. Years ago, he struggled with drinking problems, but that seems not to have reemerged during his PD.

Thomas Graboys, once a star cardiologist in Boston, is now retired from his work as a cardiologist because of the onset of PD. He lost his first wife (Caroline) to cancer just a few years before he was diagnosed with PD. In addition, Graboys' form of PD involves a severe form of Lewy body disease, and thus he is also dealing with progressively worsening dementia. Graboys (and we along with him) rages against his PD, his dementia, and all of his other losses. His memoirs (Graboys & Zheutlin, 2008) give us detailed accounts of his efforts to resist depression and, with the help of a psychotherapist, to funnel his rage and grief away from his loved ones and his caretakers and onto God or the fates. Over and over in his memoirs, Graboys broods over the effects of the disease on his primary relationships, especially with his wife. Among the many neuropsychiatric problems PD patients have to contend with, one of the most searing is their anxiety. Notably, the anxiety is most often about becoming a burden on their families. Graboys lays out all of the dilemmas, frustrations, hopes, and fears he has for every relationship in his life—from those with his former patients to those with his grandchildren, and especially for that with his wife, Vicki. Graboys displays a fierce determination to prevent the disease from defining him, and thus he shows us that PD cannot be considered apart from the person it afflicts. Each case of PD is unique.

In 1987, Morton Kondracke's wife, Milly, noticed that she could not write a normal letter "K" and that her handwriting was becoming cramped. This handwriting difficulty is a very common complaint of patients with PD. It sometimes takes the form of a micrographia (i.e., very small and cramped script). Thomas Hobbes, the political philosopher mentioned above, displayed signs of micrographia until he had to turn over all his major writing tasks to his assistants after his PD progressed. At the age of 47, Milly found herself grappling with similar handwriting problems and then was eventually diagnosed with PD. Kondracke was a prominent TV political commentator and journalist. When his wife developed PD, he unfailingly gave himself to her service and then later wrote a beautiful set of memoirs (Kondracke, 2001) about her illness. Like most people with PD, she battled severe depression throughout the illness. The two of them searched desperately for a cure, going from doctor to doctor, each time having to wearily tell the story of her symptoms. Like many other patients with PD, Milly was eventually put on a huge assortment of pills that in combination were potentially lethal and, in any case, clearly affected her neuropsychiatric status. After the danger of polypharmacy was eliminated, Milly decided to undergo a 2-day-long brain surgery, including a pallidotomy, and then an implantation of a device to support DBS. Neither surgery worked for her. Throughout her battle with PD, Milly experienced multiple falls and often had to be rushed to the emergency room for stitches. As the PD progressed, she could no longer swallow properly or speak properly. They had to sell their house (at a huge loss) to move to a safer environment for Milly. Using paper letters, Milly often spelled out the words "I don't want to live like this!" and "I want to die." Milly died in 2004. Those are the bare facts of Milly's story. When I discuss the neuropsychiatric syndromes of PD in this book, it must be remembered that those syndromes happen to real people like Milly. Sometimes these people find themselves in desperate straits, trying to find some relief from a chronic illness and often undergoing new medical treatments that raise hope for a while but usually end up helping only a small minority of PD patients. The spectacular success associated with LD is, unfortunately, an all too rare medical story.

Although Pope John Paul II and Michael J. Fox have demonstrated that one can live fully with PD, the bitter reality lies somewhere between the Pope's and Fox's experiences and that of Dr. Graboys' and Milly Kondracke's experiences. There is continual loss, continual strain on family relationships, continual crises, constant temptations to depression, and constant frustration with the health care system. Despite all these challenges people with PD typically find a way to live well and even flourish. This is the context within which we will be examining the neuropsychiatric disorders of PD. We must constantly remember that we are dealing with human beings who are confronting tremendous suffering and loss on an almost daily basis. But they are also people who find ways to hold onto joys and produce new ones in their lives. They do not stop living just because of the disease. It is a remarkable fact that despite the ravages of the disease, each patient with PD never allows himself or herself to be defined by the disease. I will be arguing throughout this book that the main effect of PD with respect to its neuropsychiatric effects is an assault on the agentic aspects of the self. The agentic self is the acting self, the doing self, the self that plans, moves, searches for valued things, and attains its goals. There is an abundance of evidence for my position on the agentic self in PD, yet it must not be forgotten there is this other aspect of the self, the self that refuses to be defined by the disease, that seems not to be affected or even impaired by the disease.

I now turn to a detailed description of the clinical course of the disease.

Neuropsychiatric Disorders of PD

The neuropsychiatric symptoms of PD such as depression, apathy, anxiety, hallucinations, and psychosis characteristically appear or emerge at different stages of the disease, and they all exhibit complex relationships with the classical motor (tremor, bradykinesia, rigidity, and postural instability) deficits of the disease. For example, although depression is common even before onset of the motor symptoms, it becomes severe in the mid and late stages of the disease. Apathy is more common in later stages, whereas anxiety disorders are more common in early- and mid-stage patients. Speech act deficits appear in the early and mid stages of the diseases as well. In addition to differing as a function of stage of disease, symptoms are also influenced by side of onset of the disease. Keeping in mind the dependence of neuropsychiatric and cognitive deficits of PD on stage and side of onset of PD, I will review the natural clinical history of PD in what follows. I will conclude this chapter with a discussion of the proposed causes of PD.

Diagnostic Criteria for PD

Most scientific papers on PD use the diagnostic criteria for PD that were developed by the UK Parkinson's Disease Society Brain Bank (see table 1.2; Hughes, Daniel, Kilford, & Lees, 1992). The criteria require that the patient display slowed movement (bradykinesia) and at least one of the other three cardinal signs of PD (tremor, postural instability, and rigidity). Once these hurdles are cleared, the criteria require that other potential causes of these motor deficits be ruled out. Other potential causes include brain injury of various kinds, related disorders such as progressive supranuclear palsy, and various forms of dementing illnesses. If the motor deficits ever remitted for a sustained period of time, PD is not the likely diagnosis. Exposure to 1-methyl-4-phenyl-1,2,3,6-tetrahydropyridine (MPTP)— a drug that becomes toxic to dopamine cells when broken down in the brain and that was found in some recreational drugs back in the 1980s—can cause parkinsonism as well. Step 3 in the diagnosis involves the collection of supportive data such as unilateral signs (tremor on one side of the body, etc.) and a good response to LD therapy.

Hoehn and Yahr Rating Scale

Once a diagnosis of PD has been made, the patient can expect the disorder to get progressively worse over the duration of several years. Most patients will pass through well-known stages of the disease, termed Hoehn–Yahr stages (Hoehn & Yahr, 1967), as the disorder moves from being a largely asymmetric tremor with very few other symptoms to whole-body shakiness, postural instabilities, and significant mood and mental problems. Sometimes the patient progresses into a full-blown dementia that mimics Alzheimer's dementia, but thankfully not every patient faces this prospect.

The most widely used rating scale for stage identification is the Hoehn–Yahr scale (see table 1.3). This scale was based on clinical observations of the natural history of the disease as it occurred in hundreds of patients before the discovery of LD. It describes five general stages in PD, ranging from stage 1 (unilateral disease, limited to one side of the body) to stage 5 (wheelchair bound or bedridden unless aided).

For more detailed observations of the motor symptomatology of any given patient, neurologists use the Unified Parkinson Disease Rating Scale (Fahn, Elton, and Members of the UPDRS Development Committee, 1987; Goetz et al., 2008). This set of scales is also very often used in research on PD.

Table 1.2
UK Parkinson's Disease Society brain bank clinical diagnostic criteria

Step 1: Diagnosis of parkinsonian syndrome
• Bradykinesia (slowness of initiation of voluntary movement with progressive reduction in speed and amplitude of repetitive actions)
• And at least one of the following:
Muscular rigidity
4–6 Hz rest tremor
Postural instability not caused by primary visual, vestibular, cerebellar, or proprioceptive dysfunction.

Step 2: Exclusion criteria for PD
• History of repeated strokes with stepwise progression of parkinsonian features
• History of repeated head injury
• History of definite encephalitis
• Oculogyric crises
• Neuroleptic treatment at onset of symptoms
• More than one affected relative
• Sustained remission
• Strictly unilateral features after 3 years
• Supranuclear gaze palsy
• Cerebellar signs
• Early severe autonomic involvement
• Early severe dementia with disturbances of memory, language, and praxis
• Babinski sign
• Presence of cerebral tumor or communicating hydrocephalus on CT scan
• Negative response to large doses of LD (if malabsorption excluded)
• MPTP exposure

Step 3: Supportive prospective positive criteria for PD (three or more required for diagnosis of definite PD)
• Unilateral onset
• Rest tremor present
• Progressive disorder
• Persistent asymmetry affecting side of onset most
• Excellent response (70% to 100%) to LD
• Severe LD-induced chorea
• LD response for 5 years or more
• Clinical course of 10 years or more

Source: From Hughes, A. J., Daniel, S. E., Kilford, L., & Lees, A. J. (1992). Accuracy of clinical diagnosis of idiopathic Parkinson's disease. A clinico-pathological study of 100 cases. *Journal of Neurology, Neurosurgery, and Neuropsychiatry, 55,* 181–184. Reprinted with permission.

Table 1.3
Hoehn–Yahr (HY) Parkinson's Disease Rating Scale

Stage 1
• Signs and symptoms appear only on one side of the body.
• Symptoms are mild.
• Symptoms may be inconvenient, but they are not disabling.
• Usually a tremor is present in only one limb.
• Friends and other loved ones have noticed changes in posture, movement, and in facial expression.

Stage 2
• Symptoms appear on both sides of the body.
• Symptoms cause minimal disability.
• Posture and gait are affected.

Stage 3
• Body movements are slowed significantly.
• Symptoms cause moderately severe problems with normal functioning.

Stage 4
• Symptoms are severe.
• The individual can still walk, but only to a limited extent.
• There is rigidity and slowness of movement.
• One is no longer able to live alone.

Stage 5
• Wheelchair bound.

The Unified Parkinson's Disease Rating Scale

The Unified Parkinson's Disease Rating Scale (UPDRS; Fahn et al., 1987; Goetz et al., 2008) is a composite set of scales consisting of six sections. Each item within each section asks a trained physician or scientist to rate the patient's abilities/performance on a scale of 0 to 4 (normal to severely affected). The UPDRS takes approximately 20 to 30 minutes to administer. Part I of the UPDRS consists of four items assessing cognitive symptoms, mood, motivation, and the presence or absence of a thought disorder. Part II consists of 13 items describing difficulties on performance of a number of activities of daily living such as bathing, dressing, using utensils, and so forth. Part III is a 14-item section on tremor, assessment of facial and generalized bradykinesia, disease severity, finger tapping against the thumb, clenching and unclenching a fist, rising from a chair, and other tasks. Part IV assesses duration, severity, and timing of dyskinesias and motor fluctuations and the presence or absence of anorexia, sleep disturbance, or orthostatic hypotension. Part V is a modified version of the Hoehn–Yahr staging system, and Part VI is a disability scale estimating the degree of dependency in daily activities.

In general, controlled studies have found that when different trained physicians and technicians individually administer the UPDRS to the same patients, they generally get the same results. Interrater reliability correlations have been as high as 0.80 on most items (speech being the exception). The test–retest reliability of the UPDRS is also relatively high. Intraclass coefficients in the studies with the largest number of participants were over 0.90 for overall UPDRS score and around 0.80 for subscales. The UPDRS has been criticized for years for not adequately assessing nonmotor symptoms of PD such as sleep disturbances, cognitive deficits, anxiety, fatigue, depression, and autonomic symptoms such as impotence, orthostatic hypotension, and bladder and bowel dysfunction. A task force was convened by the Movement Disorder Society (MDS) in the early 2000s to add new items to the UPDRS to assess nonmotor deficits (Goetz et al., 2008). The task force completed its work in 2009, and the new version of the scales, the MDS-UPDRS, is available on the MDS Web site (www.movementdisorders.org). This new scale is an important positive development for people interested in the study of neuropsychiatric disorders of PD as it will allow us to more easily examine quantitative relationships between severity of motor and nonmotor (e.g., mood) symptoms of PD.

Clinical Symptoms and Course of PD

The average age of PD onset is approximately 50 to 60 years, but there are forms of PD where age of onset is below 40. Approximately 5% of patients present symptoms before the age of 40. An asymmetric resting tremor is the most common initial symptom to lead to the diagnosis, accounting for as many as 70% of cases. When patients think back as to early signs of their PD, they may point to pain in the shoulder, muscle rigidity, problems with fine motor skills like handwriting, buttoning up a shirt, sleep problems, and a general lack of energy. Controlled, large population studies where health status was followed in thousands of people over decades suggested that constipation, loss of smell (anosmia), and signs of rapid eye movement (REM) sleep behavior disorder (RBD; where people act out violent dreams in their sleep) very strongly predicted the onset of PD years later (Abbott et al., 2007). We will see later in the discussion of pathologic causes of PD that these early signs of PD may be due to cellular degeneration associated with Lewy body inclusions in the brain stems and homeostatic centers of the brains of people at risk for developing PD. Basically, the pathology that causes PD starts in the brain stem and then ascends up through the neuraxis until it reaches the cortex. Thus, the first signs of PD should be related to functions handled by the brain stem and then to functions handled by the autonomic regulatory centers of the brain.

The classic triad of symptoms of PD is tremor, rigidity, and bradykinesia, and each of these change with stage of disease (Fahn et al., 1987; Global Parkinson's Disease Survey Steering Committee, 2002; Goetz et al., 2008; Hoehn & Yahr, 1967). Many experts add a fourth symptom, gait/postural instability, to the classical triad.

Bradykinesia

Bradykinesia, or slowed movement, manifests itself in various forms such as slowed walking, reduced eye blink rates, and fewer overall movements than that of the average person. The slowed movements begin in the early stages and then in later stages the individual manifests an overall paucity of movements.. All of this points to a diminution in the power of the agentic self to initiate and implement actions. Sometimes the patient will also demonstrate reduced power in his voice so that it becomes difficult to hear. Facial expressions appear immobile or "masked." To underline the fact that the bradykinesia encompasses more than basic motor acts, the patient often exhibits problems with planning, initiating, and executing coordinated and sequential actions. Notably, bradykinesia of PD is linked with something known as *kinesia paradoxica*. Patients with severe poverty of movement can sometimes demonstrate that their capacity for movement is quite intact as when someone yells fire or when someone is about to fall. In these cases, the patient can run out of the building or catch the falling person and so forth. The problem is that the agentic self does not have enough strength to initiate and control actions. Motor programs are intact and available, but the patient has difficulty activating them and controlling them once activated. Activation and control, as we will see in another chapter, requires an intact agentic self.

What causes bradykinesia? Degree of bradykinesia is correlated with degree of cell loss in the dopaminergic striatum. The reduction in the dopaminergic signal to the basal ganglia leads to reduced activation levels in the putamen and globus pallidus (cell groups in the basal ganglia that control implementation of motor actions), thus resulting in a reduction in the muscle force produced at the initiation of movement.

Tremor

The tremor seen in PD is a rhythmic, resting tremor that occurs intermittently in one limb for a few minutes and then appears a few minutes later in another limb.

Like bradykinesia, it, too, is affected by mental phenomena: it increases when the patient is concentrating or feeling anxious. An estimated 30% of patients with PD do not have resting tremor. For patients with tremor, it usually begins in one hand and then, in later stages of the disease, it appears in both limbs. Tremor in the hand usually occurs at a frequency between 4 and 6 Hz and almost always has a "pill-rolling" phenomenology that spreads from one hand to the other. Characteristically, rest tremor disappears with action and during sleep.

Rigidity

Because the muscles in PD are constantly contracted, they eventually stretch and shorten all the muscles in the body leading to painful contractures in the hands and feet as well as in the back. These pulled muscles draw the head and neck downward, thus producing a stooped posture, poor balance, propulsion (a tendency to run forward), and falling. Rigidity is experienced by patients as muscle stiffness, soreness, or cramping. When physicians test for rigidity, they look for resistance to passive movement of a limb. The resistance to movement takes on a "cogwheel" form. All of these forms of rigidity get worse with progression of the disease.

Postural Instability and Freezing

Postural instability is the bane of PD patients and their families as it leads to falls and injuries and compromises independence. It usually occurs in later stages of the disease, and it, along with freezing of gait, is the most common cause of falls in PD. Freezing is a form of akinesia (a loss of movement) and is one of the most disabling symptoms of PD. About half of all patients with PD report freezing phenomena. It typically manifests as a sudden inability to continue walking or to initiate a movement or to close one's eyelids and so forth. This is, of course, extremely dangerous when one is crossing a busy street facing oncoming traffic. Notably, patients often develop tricks to overcome freezing attacks such as imagining a line on the floor and using that to move forward or marching to an internal musical beat, and so forth. The basic idea is to use some external salient stimulus to help control movement because the internal control of movement is lost.

Nonmotor Features of PD

Nonmotor deficits of PD include autonomic dysfunction, pain and sensory abnormalities, cognitive/neurobehavioral disorders, and sleep abnormalities. Because the rest of this book is about the neurobehavioral abnormalities of PD, I will mention the autonomic abnormalities only here. In addition to the primary motor problems of PD, patients are afflicted with a host of other symptoms that are due to loss of normal autonomic nervous system (ANS) function, which in turn may be due to loss of dopamine innervation to ANS regulatory control centers. Some of these problems include constipation, sluggish bladder, decreased sexual libido, anosmia, hot flashes or chills, edema, seborrhea, excessive sweating, conjunctivitis, swallowing difficulties, and many other symptoms besides. These various afflictions need to be kept in mind when one considers the ability of PD patients to cope with the neuropsychiatric disorders of PD.

Pain in PD

Although it is clear that a majority of patients with PD report significant pain at all stages of the disease (Drake, Harkins, & Qutubuddin, 2005; Goetz, Tanner, Levy, Wilson, & Garron, 1986), it is unclear to what extent pain disturbances are due to or shaped by mood disturbances or to more central pain processing abnormalities (Djaldetti et al., 2004; Snider, Fahn, Isgreen, & Cote, 1976). In a recent study (McNamara, Stavitsky, Harris, Szent-Imrey, & Durso, 2010), we found significantly greater pain intensity ratings in PD than in control participants. All of the McGill Pain Questionnaire (Melzack, 1975) subscale scores in a left-onset PD (LPD) group were significantly related to overall mood dysfunction, but this was not the case for the right-onset PD (RPD) group. The associations between mood and pain in the LPD group were quite striking, reaching an almost perfect correlation. In addition, we found some evidence for differing expression of other pain symptoms among PD patients as a function of side of motor symptom onset. Patients with left-onset disease and greater right hemispheric pathology reported greater amounts of present pain intensity than that of control participants. Thus, we have clear evidence that one of the most disabling nonmotor symptoms of PD is related to higher control centers in the central nervous system (CNS). There is some evidence in the literature suggesting that impairment in right forebrain systems may lead to enhanced pain perception. The prefrontal cortex is known to be involved in descending pain inhibitory systems (Borckardt et al., 2007), and dopaminergic dysfunction in right forebrain neural networks may impair prefrontal inhibitory functions as well, thus resulting in increased pain perception. Notably, 15 minutes of left prefrontal repetitive transcranial magnetic stimulation decreases pain perception in healthy adults (Borckardt et al., 2007).

Having briefly reviewed the clinical course of PD, I turn now to a consideration of the causes of PD.

Causes of PD

Oxidative Stress

One of the normal consequences of biochemical processes in our bodies is the production of free radicals. These are reactive oxygen species that can damage cells in myriad ways. Mitochondria produce these and also handle them. However, mitochondria may be one of the sites of pathology in PD, and thus free radicals build up over time in persons at risk for PD. They tend to accumulate in sites that engage in a lot of metabolic work like the pigmented cells of the substantia nigra; thus, the pigmented cells of the substantia nigra are particularly vulnerable to oxidative stress and cell damage.

Environmental Toxins

A large number of epidemiologic studies have indicated that rates of PD are higher in areas where exposure to environmental toxins is a risk. Exposure to pesticides, carbon monoxide, heavy metals, or toxins in the food supply may cause damage to vulnerable CNS sites like the substantia nigra. A recent study (Costello, Cockburn, Bronstein, Zhang, & Ritz, 2009) investigated the effects of exposure to the pesticide maneb and the herbicide paraquat. The researchers found that persons who lived within 500 meters of fields sprayed with either of these two agents between 1974 and 1999 had a 75% increased risk for developing PD.

Whether the proximate cause of PD is exposure to toxins or oxidative stress, it is now understood that certain genes increase vulnerability to the disease as well.

Genetics of PD

Approximately 5% to 10% of patients with PD have a familial pattern of inheritance, and to date, linkage has been reported with 11 different genes (see table 1.4). Familial PD has been described in association with mutations in *alpha-synuclein*, ubiquitin carboxy-terminal hydrolase L1 (*UCH-L1*), *parkin*, *DJ-1*, PTEN-induced kinase 1 (*PINK1*), *LRRK2* (leucine-rich repeat kinase 2), and, more recently, in the genes encoding for Omi/HtrA2 and ATP13A2. Even patients with sporadic PD who have typical clinical and pathologic features with no family history are often found to have LRRK2 mutations. Many of these genes impact, in one way or another, the metabolic processing of protein manufacture and degradation. For example, alpha-synuclein clumps, or aggregates, called protofibrils, cause cell membrane (including mitochondrial membrane) destruction and eventual cell

Table 1.4
Genes linked to PD

Locus	Gene/Protein	Inheritance Pattern	Clinical Phenotype
PARK1	SNCA/α-synuclein	Autosomal dominant	Mid-age onset (45–60 years with typical PD ± dementia)
PARK2	PARK2/parkin	Autosomal recessive	Juvenile (<20 years) onset with atypical features
PARK3	Unknown	Autosomal dominant	Typical PD
PARK5	UCH-L1	Autosomal dominant	Mid-age onset with typical PD
PARK6	PINK1	Autosomal recessive	Early onset (20–45 years) PD with slow progression
PARK7	PARK7/DJ-1	Autosomal recessive	Early onset PD with slow progression
PARK8	LRRK2/dardarin	Autosomal dominant	Mid-age onset with typical PD ± dementia and amyotrophy
PARK10	Unknown	Genetic susceptibility	Typical PD
PARK11	Unknown	Genetic susceptibility	Typical PD
FTDP-17	MAPT/tau	Autosomal dominant	Parkinson's associated with frontotemporal dementia
SCA2	ATXN2/ataxin-2	Autosomal dominant	Typical PD
SCA3	ATXN2/ataxin-3	Autosomal dominant	Typical PD
Nurr1	NR4A2/NURR1	Likely autosomal dominant	Typical PD
Synphilin-1	SNCAIP/synphilin-1	Likely autosomal dominant	Typical PD
Mitochondria	NADH complex 1	Mitochondrial inheritance (maternal line)	Typical PD

Source: Modified from Butler and McNamara (2011, in press).

death. These alpha-synclein-related proteinaceous inclusions may be a major source of Lewy body deposition in cells in the CNS. Lewy bodies are one of the hallmark pathognomic features of PD (see below). Alpha-synuclein production is enhanced in tandem with high levels of oxidative stress as well. All of this points to the idea that cell death in the substantia nigra in PD is due, ultimately, to genetic defects that lead to failure to dispose of protein aggregates and breakdown in degradation of these aggregates through the ubiquitin/proteasome pathway. These biochemical failures that lead to protein clumps result, ultimately, in Lewy body inclusions in various cell groups in the CNS, including the striatal dopamine groups. The Lewy body inclusions disrupt cellular functions and then the cells die off.

Neuropathology and Progression of PD
Braak and colleagues (Braak, Ghebremedhin, Rüb, Bratzke, & Del Tredici, 2004) proposed that the varying degrees of synuclein pathology follow a definite sequence

Table 1.5
Pathologic stages of PD proposed by Braak and colleagues

Stage 1: Medulla oblongata and olfactory bulb lesions in dorsal nucleus of cranial nerves IX and X. Intermediate reticular formation, olfactory bulb, and anterior olfactory nuclei.

Stage 2: Pontine tegmentum pathology of stage 1 plus lesions in caudal raphe in n. gigantocellular reticular nucleus and coeruleus-subcoeruleus complex.

Stage 3: Midbrain pathology of stage 2 plus lesions in pars compacta of substantia nigra.

Stage 4: Basal prosencephalon and mesocortex pathology of stage 3 plus prosencephalic lesions, anteromedial temporal mesocortex and allocortex (CA-2 plexus).

Stage 5: Neocortex pathology of stage 4 plus lesions in prefrontal cortex and sensory association neocortical areas.

Stage 6: Neocortex pathology of stage 5 plus lesions in first-order sensory association cortex, premotor cortex, and primary sensory and motor cortex.

Source: Modified from Braak, H., Ghebremedhin, E., Rüb, U., Bratzke, H., & Del Tredici, K. (2004). Stages in the development of Parkinson's disease-related pathology. *Cell and Tissue Research*, *318*(1), 121–134.

of stages (see table 1.5). In their proposed schema, PD pathology progresses through six stages, spreading from the medulla (stage 1) to the pons and upper brain stem (stages 2 to 3), to the anterior temporal mesocortex (stage 4), and then to the neocortex (stages 5 to 6). In short, when the synuclein pathology reaches stage 3 or 4, pathology involves the substantia nigra and other midbrain structures.

Neuropathologic studies of PD suggest that clinical signs of PD begin to emerge when the ventrolateral region of the substantia nigra has lost greater than 60% of its neurons due to synuclein pathology. Clinical, pathology, and neuroimaging studies all suggest that the neuropathologic process begins approximately 5 years before the clinical onset of symptoms.

The progression of PD, however, may be nonlinear, with a more rapid rate of decline in early disease and slower progression later, or vice versa, with rapid decline later and steady decline initially. Only empirical work will resolve this issue. The Deprenyl and Tocopherol Antioxidant Therapy of Parkinsonism (DATATOP, 1996) study enrolled 800 subjects with early (Hoehn–Yahr stage 1 and 2) untreated PD patients. Three hundred fifty-three of these patients were treated with placebo or placebo plus tocopherol, which was found to be ineffective. Overall, the total UPDRS score in these individuals worsened by 14% per year (approximately 4 points), and the motor portion of the UPDRS score worsened by 9% per year (approximately 2.5 points).

And finally, there is one last clinical factor that we need to discuss to understand the neuropsychiatric disorders of PD: asymmetric side of onset.

Asymmetry in PD

The motor symptoms of PD initially present predominately on one side of the body, and though poorly understood, this asymmetric disease profile may significantly influence survival rates of PD patients (Elbaz et al., 2003), response profiles to LD (Dethy et al., 1998), and risk for development of neuropsychiatric syndromes and dementia (Amick, Grace, & Chou, 2006; Direnfeld et al., 1984; Djaldetti, Ziv, & Melamed, 2006; Kaaisenen et al., 2001; Starkstein, Mayberry, Leiguarda, Preziosi, & Robinson, 1992; Tomer & Aharon-Peretz, 2004; Tomer, Levin, & Weiner, 1993). The prognostic utility of asymmetric disease profiles (e.g., the presence and magnitude of asymmetric disease presentation), in short, may be considerable. Yet, very little work has been done on the prognostic utility or clinical correlates of asymmetric disease in PD. Animal models have shown asymmetric behavior to be associated with an imbalance of neostriatal dopamine content. Single photon emission computed tomography (SPECT) and positron emission tomography (PET) studies in humans, furthermore, have consistently demonstrated correlations between reduced striatal and prefrontal dopaminergic activity contralateral to the clinically more affected side and the motor, mood, and cognitive functions associated with that side of the brain (reviewed in Djaldetti et al., 2006).

Recent epidemiologic and prevalence studies, using rigorous measurement criteria to define asymmetry, have demonstrated that between 50% and 60% of cases of PD evidence marked asymmetry of at least three motor symptoms throughout the course of the disorder. Uitti, Baba, Whaley, Wszolek, and Putzke (2005) reported that disease duration, age at onset, and left-handedness were significantly associated with asymmetric disease. That is, shorter symptomatic disease duration was associated with a greater degree of asymmetric disease, an earlier age at disease onset was associated with a greater degree of overall asymmetry, and left-handed individuals tended to have more severe disease on the left side of the body. Whereas the first two correlates (shorter duration and early age at onset) could be explained by supposing that as PD progresses symptoms become more bilaterally distributed, the link with left-handedness is more difficult to explain. Notably, Biary and Koller (1985) reported a higher incidence of left-handedness in patients with essential tremor relative to that of age-matched controls. Uitti et al. (2005) suggested that the reserve of dopamine levels in the right hemisphere (controlling the left hand) of left-handed individuals is not as high as the reserve of right-hemisphere dopamine in right-handed individuals. But, this theory would predict more severe disease on the left side of the body for both left- and right-handed individuals. Thus, the handedness correlate remains a mystery.

The primary pathology of PD is loss of midbrain dopaminergic cells. If we therefore wish to understand neuropsychiatric disorders of PD including the impact of PD on the self, then we will need to examine how dopamine supports neurocognitive processing. In what follows, I will review those aspects of forebrain dopaminergic activity that supports executive control systems that are in service to the agentic self. This will allow us to begin to explore the neuropsychiatric disorders of PD in terms of changes in executive control or the agentic self. The nature, structure, and functions of the agentic self are explicated in great detail in the following chapters. I will show that dopaminergic activity supports a goal-directed learning process (key for agentic self functions) based on prediction of reward and reinforcing stimuli—all processes crucial for choice, valuation, and agentic control more generally. In addition, I will show that striatal-prefrontal and mesocortical dopaminergic systems also support abilities to delay gratification in favor of some larger future reward (i.e., temporal discounting, another crucial piece of agentic control). Then I will show that these same dopamine systems are required for implementation of an array of executive cognitive functions (ECFs) including the central ECF called working memory. Agentic, or executive control, functions would be impossible without a working memory system that allows the agent to weigh simultaneously several options in pursuit of strategic goals. I will conclude the chapter with a summary of the dopaminergic mediation of personality traits such as extraversion and novelty-seeking behaviors that compose the agentic portions of the self system.

Dopaminergic Anatomy and Physiology

Dopaminergic afferents originate in the midbrain substantia nigra and ventral tegmental area and then innervate widespread neocortical sites including the striatum,

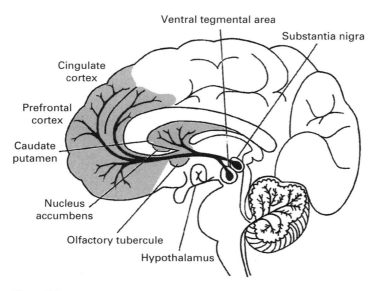

Ventral tegmental area

Substantia nigra

Cingulate
cortex

Prefrontal
cortex

Caudate
putamen

Nucleus
accumbens

Olfactory tubercule

Hypothalamus

Figure 2.1
Dopaminergic pathways of the brain. (From Fuster, J. M. 2008. *The Prefrontal Cortex*. 4th ed.
Boston: Academic Press. Copyright © 2008, Elsevier. Used with permission.)

the limbic system, the basal ganglia, and the prefrontal cortex (PFC) (see figure 2.1).
Notably, within the prefrontal regions dopamine activity is greatest in the precentral
primary motor area and then the supplementary motor area (SMA) (Fuster, 2008;
Lewis, Campbell, Foote, & Morrison, 1986). This concentration of dopamine in the
motor control regions along with the abundant evidence of dopaminergic regulation
of executive control systems (reviewed later) within the dorsolateral and medial
prefrontal regions strongly supports the idea that dopaminergic activity within the
prefrontal regions supports agentic aspects of the self and that PD represents a loss
of this agentic self.

The sources of prefrontal dopamine lie within three major nuclei of the midbrain,
sometimes designated as A8 (the retrorubral area), A9 (the substantia nigra pars
compacta; SNc), and A10 (the ventral tegmental area; VTA) (Oades & Halliday,
1987; Voorn, Vanderschuren, Groenewegen, Robbins, & Pennartz, 2004). The
ascending dopaminergic SNc pathway projects mostly to the (dorsal) caudate
nucleus and putamen (collectively called the neostriatum) and is generally referred
to as the nigrostriatal pathway. Thus, the nigrostriatal pathway primarily, though
not exclusively, supports motor and indirectly (via projections from caudate to

PFC) prefrontal functions. By contrast, the dopaminergic afferents from the VTA project to the nucleus acccumbens circuit and other limbic regions such as the amygdala, bed nucleus of stria terminalis, cingulate cortex (including the anterior cingulate cortex, or ACC, a site important for conflict monitoring), and portions of the hippocampal complex. A mesocortical projection from the VTA projects primarily to frontal portions of the neocortex such as the dorsolateral prefrontal cortex (DLPFC) as well as the supplementary motor (SMA) and premotor regions.

There are a series of major motor, motivational, and cognitive circuits that are targets of the ascending dopaminergic systems. I will just briefly mention these major systems here insofar as they overlap with dopaminergic anatomy (see table 11.1 in chapter 11). The striatum is a set of interrelated subcortical structures called the caudate, the putamen, and the nucleus accumbens circuit (NAC). The caudate is densely interconnected with dorsal regions of the PFC and thus supports ECFs. The putamen appears to support motor programming and thus is clearly implicated in the production of the motor symptoms of PD. The NAC is densely interconnected with limbic system sites and is therefore implicated in a variety of mood disorders, addiction, and other neuropsychiatric disorders. The basal ganglia includes the striatum along with the globus pallidus (a motor output region) and the subthalamic nucleus (a relay to PFC).

There are two major families of dopamine (DA) receptors: the D_1-like family (D_1 and D_5) and the D_2-like family (D_2, D_3, and D_4). Activation of D_1 receptors heightens the signal-to-noise ratio of cell responsiveness, suppressing firing in relatively hyperpolarized cells and expediting firing in relatively depolarized ones. Some of the D_2 receptors are autoreceptors that, when stimulated, act to inhibit DA release. Each of the two receptor types is affected in different ways by a pool of extracellular DA that affects background or baseline levels of tonic dopaminergic activity. In the primate neocortex, both D_1 and D_2 receptors are present, with highest concentrations in the frontal lobe, but D_1 is about 10–20 times more frequent than D_2 (Lidow, Goldman-Rakic, Gallager, & Rakic, 1991).

Tonic versus Phasic Mechanisms of DA Release

Some DA cells appear to be driven by an endogenous "pacemaker" mechanism such that they maintain a constant level of background dopaminergic activity (Bunney, Chiodo, & Grace, 1991; Grace, 2002). These tonically active DA cells yield a constant level of dopaminergic activity in the CNS and appear to be correlated with the subjective sense of vigor or restlessness. In addition to these tonically active DA cells, there are other DA cells that tend to fire in bursts. This "phasic" dopaminergic activity appears to be especially important for neurobehavioral functions including higher cognitive processing. Phasic signaling occurs when DA neurons fire action potentials in synchronized bursts of three to six action potentials every 100 milliseconds or so. These phasic bursts are believed to increase extracellular DA transiently at sites to which DA axons project.

It is not clear how tonic DA is related to phasic dopaminergic activity. It may be that tonic and phasic signaling patterns sometimes act in opposing ways with one inhibiting or regulating the other. But for most operations, it appears that tonic activity is necessary for and supports phasic bursts and vice versa. The picture, however, is complex. It may be that tonic activity can only benefit phasic activity when DA release is mediated via glutamatergic activity. Both in the striatum (Grace, 1991) and in the PFC (Takahata & Moghaddam, 1998), glutamatergic receptors on the DA cell axon terminals regulate release of DA from these terminals, but such release seems to depend on some baseline background tonic activity.

With respect to neuropsychiatric disorders of PD, if tonic activity reciprocally regulates phasic activity via glutamatergic or other mechanisms, then reduced baseline extracellular tonic DA activity would have the effect of disinhibiting phasic DA action, thus yielding abnormal cognitive processes possibly leading to ECF deficit and possibly even delusional belief systems. Conversely, an increase in the background tonic level of DA in the striatum (e.g., via use of CNS suppressants) may yield downregulation of phasic dopaminergic activity and thus poverty of cognitive content. The latter sometimes occurs in apathy syndromes of PD.

The Temporal Difference Algorithm

Decades of investigation into the neurophysiologic properties of midbrain DA neurons suggests that some proportion of DA neurons fires at a rate proportional to whether an expected reward was greater than or less than expected (Schultz, 1998). An unexpected large reward elicits enhanced firing, and a disappointing reward dampens firing. Thus, dopaminergic firing patterns are proportional to the prediction error ($\delta t = V_{stimulus} - V_{baseline}$) of the temporal difference (TD) algorithm so that positive δt corresponds with neuronal excitation and negative δt corresponds with inhibition.

Sutton and Barto (1990, 1998) pointed out that a great deal of adaptive learning can take place if one follows the following three-step procedure: (1) predict the consequences of the value to you of implementing some action or choice you are considering; (2) after ranking the available options/candidate actions, choose the action with the highest predicted value or ranking; and (3) update the accuracy of that prediction by computing the difference between what you predicted and what actually happened. Note that step 1 can be successful to the extent that one has the ability to simulate mentally a variety of potential consequences associated with a variety of potential actions. This simulation ability is sometimes called counterfactual processing. I will have more to say about processing of counterfactual simulations in the chapter on cognitive deficits in PD (chapter 5).

This three-step adaptive learning algorithm has come to be called the TD algorithm in the computational neuroscience literature, and interestingly enough, it is a specialty of dopaminergic signaling. The TD mechanism builds on the Rescorla–Wagner model of reinforcement learning and conditioning. Rescorla and Wagner (1972) argued that the associative strength of conditioned stimuli is a function of an error-correcting learning rule that was in turn driven by the magnitude of the discrepancy between an unexpected and an expected outcome. Thus, learning happens best when events are not predicted or when there is a near-miss in the prediction. Too great an error makes it difficult to adjust the parameters of the simulation in order to make a better prediction next time. The TD algorithm extends the Rescorla–Wagner model by capturing effects of stimuli that are extended across arbitrarily defined temporal intervals. Recall that natural selection works by building on cumulative results of past selection events. In the case of organisms, those past selection events are embodied in the body and behaviors of the organisms. Adaptation is not possible unless the aim is to match a target. With a target, you can then reduce the distance between you and the target.

The TD mechanism is basically a reward-prediction error signal that carries information about timing and intensity of an expected or future reward (Houk, Adams, & Barto, 1995; Montague, Dayan, & Sejnowski, 1996; Schultz, 1998; Schultz, Dayan, & Montague, 1997). It uses the computed difference between the expected and the actual outcome to improve future outcomes. The expectation is updated based on the historical success of the stimulus to predict reward. The magnitude of the predicted award is scaled against the predicted probability of reward, thus capturing expected value of the reward. The weights of the predictive stimuli are updated when the predictions fail to match the expectations. The prediction error signal equates to the time derivative of the reward expectancy. Phasic dopaminergic activity precisely patterns with the error term in the computation such that the phasic signal increases when the reward was better than expected, decreases when the reward failed to match expectations, and does not change when the reward was as expected.

Role of Temporal Discounting in DA Signaling

The TD theory of the DA response (Houk et al., 1995; Montague et al., 1996; Schultz et al., 1997) involves modeling a time-stamped iterative process that can be thought of as an attempt to approximate the true value of some future expected reward relative to an expected cumulative discounted future reward. Because all rewards are essentially delayed rewards, it should be pointed out that the TD algorithm can be modified to account for temporal discounting of future rewards. In that case, the DA signal would modulate in proportion to the expected sum of *discounted* future rewards; that is, the signal would be attenuated in proportion to the rate at which the individual discounts future rewards (as not worth much more than immediate small or large rewards). To the extent that the modified TD algorithm can take into account the steepness of the temporal discounting curve for any given individual, it would be equivalent to the matching law from behavioral theory (Rachlin & Green, 1972). The matching law predicts that people will differ in the extent to which they will value future larger rewards relative to smaller immediate rewards. The matching law stipulates that the choice between two options is directly proportional to the relative amount of reward and inversely proportional to the relative delay of reward. It is not surprising that both animals and people *to some extent* prefer immediate rewards to delayed rewards, even when the delayed rewards are larger. Of course, the crucial question is exactly when people are able to set aside short-term rewards for longer-term gains. People differ in their ability to opt for long-term rewards over immediately available short-term rewards. To date, no hard and fast rules can predict when someone will set aside short-term rewards for their longer-term interests. That people and animals can do this is obvious. The available neurophysiologic work on temporal discounting suggests that, once again, dopaminergic activity is the crucial signaling system with respect to capturing individual differences in temporal discounting (Ross, Sharp, Vuchinich, & Spurrett, 2003).

Note that the prediction-error theory of DA signaling effects suggests that dopaminergic neurons, when firing, phasically summate inputs from all relevant dopaminergic cell groups [including prefrontal cortex, the SMA, NAC, the central nucleus of the amygdala, the habenula (a cell group connected to the retina and pineal systems), and the striatum, and so forth] to compute a temporal difference reward prediction error. The DA signal provides its target innervation regions with a signal that controls or regulates learning of optimal choices based on previous trial-and-error learning sequences. The signal to the PFC helps to train prefrontal cognitive systems to make better predictions in the cognitive realm, and the signal to the basal ganglia and motor output regions helps to train the system to better control action sequences and to improve motor learning.

Recent work from Niv and colleagues (Niv, Daw, Joel, & Dayan, 2007) suggests that the net rate of rewards received by an organism quantifies the opportunity cost of time. They further argue that this quantity is represented by tonic levels of DA in the striatum.

In summary, the available data suggest that phasic DA signals may signal reward prediction error, which can be used for reinforcement learning (Hollerman & Schultz, 1998; Schultz et al., 1997; Suri, 2002; Waelti, Dickinson, & Schultz, 2001). When an organism is not expecting a reward and it receives one, there is a positive prediction error and a burst is signaled. In contrast, when the organism is expecting a reward and it is omitted, there is a negative prediction error and there is a diminution in phasic bursts. On the other hand, the net rate of rewards received may be represented by tonic DA signaling.

PD ECF Deficits and the Diminution of Phasic Signaling

Executive cognitive functions, or ECFs, refer to such functions as planning, initiation, attention, monitoring, and adjustment of nonroutine and goal-directed behaviors. ECF dysfunction is typically mild in early PD involving a generalized slowing of cognitive processing speed (bradyphrenia) and subtle deficits in attention and working memory (Lange, Paul, Robbins, & Marsden, 1993; Lees & Smith, 1983; Levin, Llabre, & Weiner, 1989; Owen et al., 1992; Taylor & Saint-Cyr, 1992, 1995). As the disease progresses, however, these ECF deficits become more severe, with effects on control of retrieval and attentional strategies, planning, and inhibitory power. PD patients also perform abnormally on ECF tests that reliably index frontal dysfunction such as tests of planning (e.g., the Tower of London), cognitive inhibition (e.g., the Stroop Color-Word Interference Test), and verbal and semantic fluency tasks (generative word fluency) (Bayles et al., 1996; Dubois, Boller, Pillon, & Agid, 1991; McNamara & Durso, 2000; Piccirilli, D'Alessandro, Finali, Piccinin, & Agostini, 1989; Troster & Woods, 2003; Wolters & Scheltens, 1995). It is very likely that ECFs, in general, are supported by phasic DA signaling in the PFC. That phasic signaling, of course, is constrained by, influences, and interacts with basal extracellular DA stores that produce some level of tonic DA activity in the PFC.

One way to assess directly the impact of DA on ECFs in PD is to examine the impact of ingestion of LD on performance on ECF tests. LD, of course, is the major medication used by most patients with PD to increase CNS levels of DA. When ingested, LD is converted to DA and then further metabolized to norepinephrine (NE) in catecholaminergic cells containing dopamine beta-hydroxylase.

DA is converted to homovanillic acid (HVA) and NE to 3-methoxy-4-hydroxyphenylglycol (MHPG) by a combination of MAO-B and COMT. Metabolites rather than the parent neurotransmitters are frequently used as indicators of neurotransmitter activity because these metabolites tend to be more stable than their parent compounds.

Many investigators have documented strong correlations between cerebrospinal fluid homovanillic acid (CSF HVA) and ECFs in PD (Kuiper & Wolters, 1995) and in schizophrenia (Amin, Davidson, & Davis, 1992). Whereas the connection between peripheral CSF HVA and central DA activity may seem to be tenuous at best, that is not the case: The link has been demonstrated to be strong. Indeed, CSF HVA has routinely been used as a marker for central dopaminergic activity (Amin et al., 1992). HVA represents the final stable metabolite of DA and closely parallels striatal dopaminergic activity after stimulation of the nigrostriatal pathway (Korf, Grasdijk, & Westerink, 1976) or pharmacologic manipulation. Without question, the dominant DA metabolite in human striatum and CSF is HVA. Analysis of CSF HVA as a marker for tissue DA is based on the fact that brain extracellular fluid is contiguous with CSF. It has been specifically demonstrated that stimulation of the nigra (producing increases in striatal DA metabolism) results in the release of HVA into CSF. In human autopsy data, strong correlations exist between ventricular CSF HVA and striatal tissue HVA concentrations (Stanley, Träskman-Bendz, & Dorovini-Zis, 1985). HVA released into ventricular CSF reaches the lumbar CSF space through well-documented CSF flow patterns (Haaxma-Reiche, Piers, & Beekhuis, 1989). Evidence of a ventricular-lumbar CSF gradient for CSF HVA as well as observations that lumbar CSF HVA levels are dramatically attenuated when ventricular-lumbar CSF flow is disrupted (Post, Kotin, & Goodwin, 1973; Wester et al., 1990) serve as evidence that lumbar CSF HVA is almost exclusively derived from the brain. Finally, some studies have linked lumbar CSF HVA to prefrontal dopaminergic activity as well, in both non-human primates (Elsworth, Leahy, Roth, & Redmond, 1987) and in humans (Weinberger, Berman, & Illowsky, 1988; Wolfe et al., 1990).

In addition to correlations between CSF HVA and ECF performance, administration of LD has been shown to improve significantly performance of PD patients on ECF tests such as the Wisconsin Card Sort Test (WCST; Kulisevsky et al., 1996; Lange et al., 1993), the Tower of London (TOL) planning test (Lange et al., 1993; Lange, Paul, Naumann, & Gesell, 1995; Owen et al., 1995), verbal fluency tasks

(Downes, Sharp, Costall, Sagar, & Howe, 1993; Gotham, Brown, & Marsden, 1988; Lange et al., 1993), and various other forms of intellectual functioning linked to ECFs (McNamara, Clark, Krueger, & Durso, 1996). These LD-induced performance changes in ECFs occur even after motor components of the tasks are eliminated or minimized. It is unknown whether these effects persist as the disease progresses. The effects of LD on ECF performance may be dose dependent such that too high or too low a dose impairs performance. In a seminal study, Gotham et al. (1988) assessed the performance of PD patients on four ECF tests that are known to be sensitive to prefrontal cortical dysfunction and found that verbal fluency was within normal limits while patients were on LD but declined significantly (at least with the alternation task) when patients were off LD. WCST performance, however, was impaired both on and off LD.

In attempting to understand the role of DA signaling in cognitive deficits of PD, we may have to assume that gradual (over the course of years) loss of stores of extracellular DA results in diminution of overall dopaminergic tone followed by the classic motor deficits of PD. As alluded to above, synchronized burst firing of dopaminergic neurons may carry the TD prediction error signal but, in addition, may have an impact on background tonic DA activity by transiently increasing extracellular stores of DA. Regardless of the effects of PD on extracellular DA and tonic DA, recent evidence also suggests that PD has a differential effect on phasic DA signaling (Sandberg & Phillips, 2009). A gradual diminution in strength of phasic signaling is theorized to occur initially in the dorsal striatum (putamen), then in the caudate, then the NAC, and the PFC. But, this schema does not seem to capture adequately the very early appearance of personality changes and ECF deficits in de novo PD patients. Whatever the course of DA signaling decline in PD, it is clearly a crucial causative factor in mental dysfunction of PD.

The Interaction of Phasic and Tonic DA Signaling

There is direct evidence that the interaction of the phasic and tonic signaling systems directly influences higher cognitive functions like working memory. A host of physiologic, cognitive, and pharmacologic studies has established the fact that prefrontally linked working memory systems require an optimum level of dopaminergic activity to function properly. DA appears to be crucial for ECFs at the cognitive level as well. Brozoski, Brown, Rosvold, & Goldman (1979) showed that pharmacologically depleting the PFC of DA stores (in rhesus monkeys) led to severe deficits on executive function tasks (spatial delayed alternation). Too much or too little DA activity impairs working memory performance (Goldman-Rakic, Muly, & Williams, 2000; Mattay et al., 2000; Williams & Goldman-Rakic, 1995). The precise tuning of neural firing in the PFC with the maximum signal-to-noise in system is obtained when D_1 receptor stimulation is intermediate. One influential network model of inverted-U performance effects in the PFC is the dual-state theory of prefrontal cortex DA function proposed by Durstewitz and Seamans (Durstewitz & Seamans, 2008;). Based on neurocomputational simulations of the currents resulting from the interaction of dopamine D_1- and D_2-class receptors, the authors suggested that the optimum-range state is provided by background extracellular (i.e., tonic) D_1 receptor stimulation. This background level of activity works to maintain information stores but does not integrate new information into the system. High levels of DA phasic signaling promote the establishment of a more transient, D_2-dominated network state that is characterized by a net reduction in inhibition, thus opening the gates to the influx of new information.

Deficits in working memory and selective attention may arise from a predominately D_2-controlled network state that destabilizes the system, prevents stable short-term memories from guiding behaviors, favors distractibility, and outputs only partially formed cognitive products that are experienced as hallucinations and delusions. In contrast, if phasic signaling is impaired and the individual has to rely mostly on a very strong D_1 state, then we can expect repetition of whatever thoughts are in the system to start with (perseveration) and an inability to switch into new streams of thought. Agency, in general, would be impaired given that action selection and initiation would have to overcome the locked-in D_1 state. Thus, perturbations in the interaction of phasic and tonic DA signaling systems, as well as the TD learning algorithm, could also influence high-level regulatory structures like the agentic self in PD.

DA and Agentic Personality Styles

The personality trait *extraversion*, which appears to be composed largely of a high *agency* factor, is supported mainly by dopaminergic systems (see reviews in Canli, 2006; Depue, 2006; Knutson & Bhanji, 2006). The personality trait *novelty seeking* also seems to draw heavily on mesolimbic DA systems (Leyton et al., 2002). In our studies of personality change in PD patients (McNamara, Durso, & Harris, 2008), we have found that midstage patients tend to score higher than controls on harm-avoidance scales and lower than controls on novelty-seeking scales. Menza and colleagues (Menza, Mark, Burn, & Brooks, 1995) reported a significant correlation in a sample of midstage PD patients between novelty seeking and [18F]fluorodopa uptake in the left caudate. Kaasinen et al. (2001), in contrast, reported that the novelty-seeking personality trait did not significantly correlate with [18F]fluorodopa uptake in any of the brain regions they studied. Instead, they found a highly significant positive correlation between right caudate [18F]fluorodopa uptake and a *harm-avoidance* trait in their sample of 47 PD patients. More recently, Tomer and Aharon-Peretz (2004) reported that patients with greater DA loss in the left hemisphere evidenced reduced novelty seeking whereas patients with reduced DA in the right hemisphere reported higher harm avoidance than that of matched healthy controls. This set of results makes sense if harm avoidance can be thought of as the flip side of extraversion or novelty-seeking behaviors.

Personality traits of extraversion, harm avoidance, novelty seeking, and the like may all be influenced by genetically determined levels of tonic DA as well. These background levels of tonic DA, in turn, interact with exogenously introduced drugs to shift transiently personality styles as well as agentic control functions. In people with high baseline DA levels, administration of a drug like bromocriptine will impair reward sensitivity (and enhance punishment sensitivity) by reducing DA release via modulation of presynaptic D_2 receptors. Conversely, in the low-DA subjects, bromocriptine will enhance reward sensitivity and decrease punishment sensitivity by increasing dopaminergic transmission. Harm avoidance, whatever else it is, may be related to the inability to experience reward and an enhanced sensitivity to punishment. At the cognitive level, harm avoidance may index a reduction in the strength of the agentic self in PD. If the agentic self depends on optimum or relatively high levels of tonic DA and harm avoidance is due to a reduction in tonic DA, then harm-avoidant behavioral strategies reflect a loss of agentic control. Among other things, agentic control implies an ability to inhibit incoming noxious stimuli (i.e., to diminish sensitivity to punishment). A loss of agentic control would, therefore, increase harm-avoidance strategies.

Models of DA and PD Neuropsychiatry

How might the above-reviewed models of dopaminergic activity influence our thinking about neuropsychiatry of PD? We can model the cognitive and agentic aspects of the self in terms of DA-supported feedback and feed-forward models of action control. These models of action depend on precisely the same optimization mechanisms, or error-correction-updating procedures, that the DA TD algorithm uses. Thus, it should come as no surprise that dopaminergic activity will be central to capturing agentic aspects of the self, and this is the aspect of the self construct that is most impaired in PD. This is a crucial fact because it affects the diverse phenomenology of the neuropsychiatric disorders of PD including the personality changes, the apathy, depression, and anxiety syndromes of PD. In the latter case (anxiety), the contributing factor may be overstimulation of the limbic DA systems due to loss of descending inhibition on limbic system sites attributable to impairment in PFC due ultimately to loss of DA signal in PFC. Similarly, depression and apathy may result when the PFC and executive control system are dysfunctional. Impulsivity and loss of control are exacerbated when the executive, or agentic, self can no longer effectively inhibit limbic-based impulsive responding. The basic problem is loss of balance between PFC and subcortical limbic and basal ganglia networks. What creates the precise set of symptoms associated with each syndrome depends on where the primary dysfunction or lesion or imbalance is located.

3 The Nature and Functions of the Agentic Self

We will be examining the neuropsychiatric syndromes that one sees in PD through the lens of the agentic self. The agentic self is that component of a person's identity or unified self that makes decisions and acts. The agentic self deliberates, plans, learns, and acts. It has been called by many names including the executive self, the active self, the actor, the goal-driven self, the purpose-driven self, and many others besides (see review on self systems by Boyer, Robins, & Jack, 2005). The idea though is simple: The agentic self is that part of the self that formulates goals, makes decisions, and acts. As Bandura (2001, p. 2) summarized in his exhaustive review on the topic, "Agency embodies the endowments, belief systems, self-regulatory capabilities and distributed structures and functions through which personal influence is exercised, rather than residing as a discrete entity in a particular place." Although we cannot point to a particular place in the brain and say "There is the agentic self," we will see that it is the case that the agentic self is associated with a particular set of widely distributed neuronal networks. Those networks are distributed it is true, but it is also true that not *all* networks in the brain support agency. Instead, some networks are more crucial than others, and this fact constrains cognitive models of agency.

The agentic self system is future oriented and much less dependent on autobiographical memories than are other subcomponents of the unified self. Throughout this book, I will contrast the agentic self system with what I call the minimal self system. The minimal self system depends more strongly on autobiographical memories than does the agentic system—though both systems of course draw on memories to compute self-related operations of all kinds. Gallagher (2000) distinguishes broadly between the *minimal self* and the *narrative self*, but his narrative self is different from what I refer to as the agentic self. His minimal self, however, is very close to what I am calling the minimal self as well. The minimal self in my view is that self that is present when we are just sitting there daydreaming and feeling slightly disinhibited. It is co-extensive, however, with the sense of self that arises from bodily awareness, and thus this minimal self can also be in pain rather than in a daydreaming mood. In both Gallagher's and my minimal self, the minimal self is closely identified with and varies with bodily awareness. Its dependence on the body makes it, in my view, more prone to impulsive actions than is the case with the agentic self. For Gallagher, the minimal self also encodes a certain degree of ownership of actions and therefore of agency as well. This is not the case with my version of the minimal self. Action in my view requires a temporary suppression of passive aspects of the minimal self. I also largely identify the minimal self with the so-called "default network" composed of a set of neural structures that are active when one sits quietly, doing nothing in particular but perhaps daydreaming. We will see that that set of structures typically involves ventromedial portions of the PFC as well as an extensive set of limbic sites.

Gallagher juxtaposes his minimal self with what he calls the narrative self. The narrative self supports the self-concept I have of myself. It is the story I tell myself about the ways in which my memories are linked together to form the person that I am. I will not have much to say in this book about this aspect of the self, although it clearly informs the sense of self and the personality we experience on a daily basis. I will discuss aspects of the sense of self and personality in PD in a separate chapter.

The agentic's self identity is formed not merely from memories but rather in process, via action. Nor is the agentic self like the *reflective* aspect of the minimal self that engages in *stimulus-independent thought* or daydreaming. When, however, daydreaming morphs into model building and the online running or experimenting with these models, the agentic self makes its appearance. Mental models of possible worlds virtually always contain information on how to *act* in those possible worlds. The cognitions associated with the agentic self are largely instrumental—even the simulations of possible worlds contain specifications on prospective actions that would apply in those imaginary worlds and are done to improve prediction and goal attainment in the real world. In short, the agentic self is future oriented, goal oriented, and action oriented.

Impairment in key cognitive operations (e.g., planning, choosing, and implementing strategies directed at attainment of long-term goals) associated with the agentic self constitutes, in my view, the core cognitive impairment in PD. This impairment decisively influences the phenomenology of the neuropsychiatric syndromes in PD or so I will argue in this book. Thus, in addition to surveying systematically the cognitive phenomenology, mechanisms, and neurology of each syndrome, we will also evaluate the extent to which each syndrome can be understood as a disorder of the agentic self. In each case, we will postulate not merely a loss or diminution in processes associated with the agentic rather than any other component of the self system, but we will, in addition, attempt to identify those aspects of the agentic self that can best account for the symptoms of the psychiatric disorder itself.

To accomplish the above goals, we will need to discuss systematically the cognitive structure and processing systems associated with the agentic self. But first we will situate the agentic self within the larger framework of the various self systems and decision-making processes that have been studied by cognitive scientists.

Complexity of the Unified Self System

The sense of a unified self or a single coherent identity that is a microcosm or a complete world unto itself appears to draw on several psychological and neuropsychological domains such as autobiographical memory, emotional and evaluative systems, agency or the sense of being the cause of some action, self-monitoring, bodily awareness, mind-reading or covert mimicking of other's mental states, subjectivity or perspectivalness in perception, and finally, the sense of unity conferred on consciousness when it is invested with the subjective perspective (Churchland, 2002; Gallagher, 2000; Metzinger, 2003; Northoff & Bermpohl, 2004). It is the subjective or first-person perspective that creates the unity or the microcosmic world that we know as the self. The unified self manifests the binding problem par excellence. The binding problem refers to the feat accomplished by the mind/brain of creating a unity, a single conscious experience out of a disparate series of unrelated perceptions. The unified self weaves together disparate streams of processing and seemingly independent streams of consciousness into one thematic whole that yields a distinctive subjective *feel* or *take* on the outside world. Each person is utterly and irreducibly unique and irreplaceable. Each person carries around within him a take on the world that is his alone, and when he is gone, that perspective forever vanishes never to be replaced. Each person is an end in himself and cannot be treated as a means toward some other end. Even when a person is reduced to slavery, the victim's personhood cannot be violated or damaged without the interior consent of the victim. This is the great insight on personhood and identity provided by the stoics of the ancient world. Because the microcosm is a creation of the person himself (it is after all first person dependent) in interaction with the outside infinite (the world, the cosmos or the deity, etc.), only he can destroy it. Personhood (the microcosm) therefore is a creation of two wills: the individual himself and the outside infinite (e.g., "god" for the Stoics and Christians.) A person's internal world cannot be measured as it too is infinite, has infinite depth. Various portions of it can be described and even shared with others but it cannot (as Heraclitus said) be plumbed. The individual who has become a person has infinite space within: He has desires for the infinite, thoughts concerning the infinite and emotions that are, or border on the, ecstatic; that is, emotions about some infinite mystery, beauty, or horror. The unified self is all of these things and more. Thankfully this book is not about the unified self but about the agentic self—a much less mysterious entity but a no less impressive entity at that, even though it is a mere subcomponent of the unified self.

At a minimum, the unified self is composed of several major subcomponents or subpersonalities or subselves, each of which draws on the above cognitive processes (e.g., autobiographical memory, subjectivity, perspectivalness, bodily awareness, etc.) to a greater or lesser extent. Among these I will mention only the most important for our study. I have already mentioned the minimal or bodily self and the narrative self. There is also the relational self, that self that interacts with others in the social world. Of course the agentic self, insofar as it acts in the social world, must overlap with the relational self, and we will examine one situation where this overlap clearly occurs. That situation is the utterance or comprehension of a speech act when language is used by some speaker to accomplish a social action. Although all these selves can be treated to some extent as distinct entities, they obviously overlap in their functions to a considerable extent. The phenomenological and functional distinctions between them are fuzzy. Obviously, the bodily self draws on bodily awareness and subjectivity more than it does perspectivalness, and conversely the relational self draws on perspective-taking abilities more than it does bodily awareness, and so forth. But the relational self and the bodily self clearly must overlap functionally at some point. It is important to keep this fact in mind when considering the cognitive architecture and functions of the agentic self. I will say only a few words about each of these selves before turning to an analysis of the agentic self.

Gallagher (2000) has argued that the minimal self is composed of two bare necessities for any person: a sense of ownership of one's own body and acts and a sense of agency or the ability to cause acts to happen. The sense of agency, however, is more properly housed with a whole other self concept, that of the agentic self. Thus I would equate the minimal self with a sense of awareness and ownership of one's own body but reserve the sense of causal efficacy to the agentic self. Neuropsychological data such as the dissociation between the sense of causal efficacy of some acts versus the sense of ownership of various other acts supports this distinction. Most often of course we experience causal efficacy as giving rise to the sense of ownership of those acts as well. My only point here is that the two experiences can be dissociated and that the sense of ownership can adhere to causeless acts just as well as to caused acts, and thus bodily awareness per se belongs primarily to the minimal self whereas effortful action belongs to the agentic self.

The bodily sense of self refers to all those experiences attached to the somesthetic senses including the preeminent sense of pain. This subcomponent of the unified self can be dissociated from all other subcomponents of the self and thus is a true subcomponent of the larger unified self. You can get pain without it being part of a minimal, narrative, relational, or agentic self. That is what is interesting about pain. It can so capture consciousness that it blots out all other subcomponents of the self. In fact, pain can be controlled only when it is brought under the auspices of some other subcomponent of the unified self. The narrative self will give it meaning and therefore reduce its sting. The agentic self will use it for fuel to attain various goals and therefore reduce its sting. The relational self will use it as a strategic asset to manipulate others. The minimal self will attempt to assimilate the pain into its concept of bodily integrity, and so forth. Thus, the bodily self is special in that it can encompass the special experience of sensory pain. No other self type can do that without changing the pain sensation itself.

The relational self is the social self. It is the self in relation to others. Within the cognitive system, it is always a node that is linked with nodes representing significant social others. It makes possible, uses, and constitutes social knowledge. Mead (1934) pointed out that the relational self is shaped by how we perceive others responding to ourselves. That is, it is a social construct that arises from how we think others are thinking of us. This means that the relational self depends crucially on *theory of mind* or perspective-taking abilities or the extent to which we can accurately model the thoughts others are having about us. We shape ourselves in relation to those thoughts. In stark contrast to the unified self, the relational self can become an object for itself. Thus, paradoxically the relational self can reflect on itself only when it treats itself as an object rather than as a person or microcosm.

The narrative self is the hero or heroine in the stories we make up about ourselves. The narrative self is dependent on the language faculty and language and cognitive resources of the individual. An agentic self is often depicted in these narratives, but it is constrained by the structure of narrative itself. In narrative there is always a challenge that must be overcome by the hero or heroine, and the story is about how the hero or heroine accomplished or failed to accomplish that task. The stories we tell ourselves about ourselves will often influence the goals the agentic self formulates and then pursues. The narrative self is therefore important for the agentic self.

For example, Tom will not submit an application to the writing program because he believes the story he tells himself about his writing abilities. In contrast, Tom will submit an application to the science program even though he is not objectively qualified—again because of the story he tells himself about his abilities.

We turn now to a review of the properties of the agentic self.

Properties of the Agentic Self

To the extent that the agentic self reflects on itself, it is important to point out (along with Synofzik, Vosgerau, & Newen, 2008) that the sense of agency can be decomposed into a prereflective, largely automatically induced *feeling of agency* that occurs in tandem with voluntary motor acts and an inferentially derived *judgment of agency* that occurs when we sometimes reflect on our actions. Thus, our thinking about ourselves as agents is constrained by these automatic and effortful processes that underlie our experiences of agency. In addition, our experience of agency is constrained by the acts of other agents. That is, our agentic self emerges from interactions in the social arena with other persons. The decisions and acts of other people often determine the choices we are given and the acts we perform to fulfill goals we ourselves formulate. Nevertheless, although the self is partially socially constituted, the agentic self can also shape its own social milieu and context by choosing who to interact with and when to do so. The agentic self can formulate and implement acts that do not derive from the social context but are instead generated de novo from within. People are not merely products or creatures of the social group.

What then are the major properties of the agentic self? Following Bandura (2001), I would suggest that they are intentionality, forethought, self-reactiveness, and self-reflectiveness. I will say a few words about each of these major properties as proposed by Bandura (2001), and then I will summarize other important cognitive properties of the agentic self before concluding this chapter with a discussion of how the agentic self operates given all these major and minor cognitive properties.

Intentionality

Like consciousness itself, all actions are directed toward an object or goal—even if that goal state is a mental object imagined or simulated by the agent. Acts are about goals. Thus, the representational or semantic content of actions derives from the goals formulated by the agent. Goals are created by the agent but in turn help to define the agent. People differ in the extent to which intentional states are realized in plans of action. Some people formulate a goal and then do virtually nothing to realize that goal. In those cases, goals barely differ from vague desires. But people who more fully realize their intentional states form not only superordinate goals but also a series of subgoals (sometimes called implementation intentions) to realize the overarching superordinate goal. Thus with respect to actions, intentional states are hierarchical representational structures aimed at superordinate goals, and these representational structures guide choices and actions. It should be noted as well that intentional states are intimately linked with the sense of agency itself. Haggard and colleagues (2007) have presented an array of experimental evidence that suggests that temporal effects are crucial for production of the sense of agency. When the intention to perform an action occurs close in time (of the order milliseconds) to the actual movement, the sense of agency emerges. Haggard and colleagues call this effect *intentional binding*.

Forethought

Intentional states and the formulation of goals requires forethought—a basic human ability to escape control of immediate needs and desires and to envision future needs and desires. To plan for every eventuality is impossible, but we can plan for many if we have forethought. In general, the agentic self relies on a future time perspective to develop goals and strategies for realizing those goals. The ability to look ahead, to engage in mental time travel, to simulate possible future worlds is fundamental to the agentic self. This prospective orientation is characteristic of the agentic self. It relies less on memory and more on planning. The agentic self can also flexibly shift its time horizons from the immediate future to very-long-term time horizons. It is even conceivable (e.g., among kings or philosophers, etc.) that some men have acted to have an impact on people living thousands of years into the future. The agentic self chooses its own time horizons and acts within those time horizons.

Self-Reactiveness

To be causally efficacious, an agent needs to follow through on plans to meet goals. To do that, the agent needs to be able to learn from feedback concerning progress in implementation of goals. An agent has to engage in self-regulation. Self-regulation involves ongoing self-monitoring, corrective adjustments, and self-reactions when necessary and the placing of appropriate *implementation intentions* through each step of goal attainment. Implementation intentions are potent aids to realization of goals via use of situational cues that remind an individual to utilize prelearned strategies to resist abandonment of goals and to persist in realization efforts. Implementation intentions have been shown to have health-protective effects. It has been demonstrated repeatedly that forming an implementation intention enhances many health-protective behaviors including stop-smoking efforts, cancer checks, exercise regimens, dietary changes, and even safe driving practices (Cohen & Gollwitzer, 2007).

Implementation intentions heighten the accessibility of anticipated situational cues that are often used by individuals to halt an impulsive choice, reconnect to an original superordinate goal, and "go" with a longer-term behavioral plan (Gollwitzer, 1990, 1993, 1999; Gollwitzer & Moskowitz, 1996; Gollwitzer & Schaal, 1998). For example, if you are a teenager and your superordinate goal is "I want to avoid sexually transmitted diseases while remaining sexually active," then you can form an implementation intention concerning that superordinate goal in the following way: "If I am pressured to have unprotected sex with my boyfriend, then I will stop everything and initiate a conversation on use of condoms." The situational cue that triggers the implementation intention in this case is the pressure from the boyfriend. Implementation intentions trigger action initiation in an automatic fashion when the specified situational cues are met. The more situational cues people specify in their implementation intention (i.e., the more "if" statements that people generate in their cognitive representations of their implementation intentions), and the greater the number of strategies for performing the behavior that people generate (i.e., the more "then" statements that people generate in their implementation intention), the more likely they will be to achieve their goal. If the teenage girl generates a lot of "if" statements such as "If my boyfriend pressures me for sex" or "If affection turns sexual" or "If I find myself uncomfortable . . .," then she has several cues she can rely on to trigger memory of the superordinate goal. If in addition to these memory aids she adds "then" statements to the "if" statements, she then has strategies she can call upon to defuse the situation into something less harmful. For example, when she adds a "then" statement to "If affection turns sexual . . . I will then tell my boyfriend to slow down several times until he complies," she clearly has a behavioral strategy she can call upon to carry her through the dangerous situation.

Self-Reflectiveness

Fundamental to ongoing monitoring of progress in goal realization is the ability to reflect on current action strategies and how well they are working. Insight into self and its abilities and weaknesses is not possible without some ability to reflect on self and its successes and failures. Indeed, self-reflectiveness is a key skill for the agentic self rather than for any of the other subcomponents of the unified self. No real decision making or choice is possible without self-awareness and self-monitoring.

The above four properties, intentionality, forethought, self-reactiveness, and self-reflectiveness, are the major cognitive properties of agency as identified by Bandura (2001). I turn now to a list of further cognitive properties that I suggest are part of the agentic self. At the end of this excursus, we will have the information we need to describe an initial hypothesis concerning the cognitive architecture and processing routines that support the agentic self.

Future Directedness

The sense of oneself as an agent is inherently tied to the here and now. Actions are accomplished in the ongoing present but of course are aimed at some future goal state. Nevertheless, the cues that guide action control are cues that are anchored in the present internal and external environments. This future-oriented characteristic of the agentic self does not mean that the agentic self does not have access to or use memories or references to the past. These memories are undoubtedly used to help make decisions, formulate plans and goals, and so forth. My point here, however, is that use of memories is constrained by and subordinated to the overall purpose of acting to attain some future goal.

Cause–Effect Folk Psychology

The theory of the agentic self assumes a kind of standard story about agent causation; that is, that agents plan actions, implement actions, and those actions have effects on others or the environment. Unlike all other objects in the universe, causal effects of agents are special in that they originate in the agentic self and can affect both the agentic self and many other events, agents, and causes in the wider universe. Most other objects in the universe do not originate causes themselves. Instead, they merely transmit forces or causes. Agents can both originate and transmit forces and causes. If I throw a ball toward the catcher, the umpire will call a strike. The umpire called a strike because I threw the pitch well. If the ball merely arrived at the catcher's mitt without an agent throwing it, the event would be merely another instance of one object (the ball) transmitting a force of certain magnitude and strength to some other object (the mitt), and so forth. The strike occurs because an agent threw the ball with a certain intent that was translated into certain spin with a certain force—an effect that came from years of training of an agentic self.

The sense of agency arises out of the coupling of internal predictions concerning effects of actions with their consequences in the real world. Wegner (2003) and Libet (1985) have challenged this commonsense folk psychology around agent causation. When Libet demonstrated that the conscious intention to perform an action (moving a finger) occurred only after an initial burst of brain activity called the *readiness potential*, which is standardly associated with premovement planning, Libet and others argued that the apparent causal power of conscious intentions to act may be merely epiphenomenal or even may be produced as a mere retroactive account to explain what actually occurred as something that was caused by an agent but in fact the agent, if we take the estimates of the subjects concerning the timing of their intentions as accurate, did nothing until after the brain was activated. Wegner called attention to the myriad cases where intentional states can be dissociated from the actions they were ostensibly "about," cases like *anarchic hand* phenomena after lesions deep to the SMA, automatisms, hypnosis, delusions of control, and experimentally induced changes in the sense of agency in which subjects project a feeling of causal responsibility onto actions they have not performed. But the fact that one can dissociate intentions and effects does not necessarily imply that the causal efficacy of conscious decision making is illusory. Just as perceptual illusions do not imply that the normal visual experience is nonveridical, illusions concerning conscious will do not call into question the efficacy of conscious willing itself. Similarly, the fact that the brain displays a readiness potential before subjects can identify the onset of their intention to move a finger may not imply that the intention to move is simply a story we tell ourselves about how movement occurs. The formulation of goals and the planning of movements to implement those goals is an ongoing process that involves very large swathes of the brain including the anterior PFC, the basal ganglia, the cerebellum, the SMA, and the motor cortex itself. When people are being asked to perform movements regularly and to make judgments about those movements, their brains will be active in formulation and planning of movements pretty much constantly, and thus the readiness potential will regularly and frequently occur as well.

Error Correction

Actions initiated by personal agents (i.e., by the agentic self) use what is called (borrowing from motor control theory) forward or predictive modeling to carry out the action. In forward modeling, actions are modeled by the agent, and their predicted effects or consequences are also modeled by the agent. Both the actions and their predicted effects are simulated and "run" by the agent. If when the action is actually carried out by the agent the predicted effects match or are congruent with what actually occurs, then the agent feels causally effective and "owns" the action. The thought is that "I caused those effects to happen." In forward modeling, motor commands are copied to a brain system (presumably a brain circuit involving basal ganglia, motor cortex, PFC, and cerebellum) that uses this information to predict the sensory effects of the movement. Actual effects are compared with the predicted effects (forward modeling is sometimes called a comparator). If they are incongruent, the degree of error can be used by the system to make corrections, thus improving motor and action control. As discussed in the chapter on DA (chapter 2), midbrain DA neurons instantiate this sort of error signal in their firing patterns. The signal is passed to the sites innervated by dopaminergic afferents (from the striatum and basal ganglia up to the PFC), and thus reward learning can be used to improve motor and action control. In PD of course this forward-modeling, DA-supported error-correction system is impaired. This system operates as the core of the agentic self and that is why it is reasonable to think of the nonmotor deficits of PD as an impairment in the system of the agentic self (see figure 3.1).

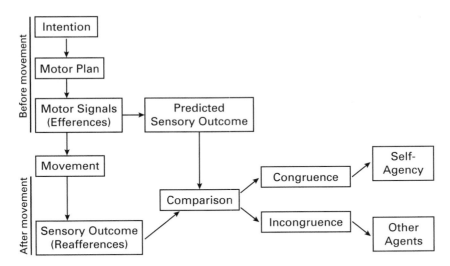

Figure 3.1
Comparator model of agentic self. When there is a congruence between predicted and actual events, a sense of agency emerges. When there is mismatch between predicted and actual events, agency may be ascribed to others—especially when the individual is cognitive impaired (From David, N., Newen, A., & Vogeley, K. 2008. The "sense of agency" and its underlying cognitive and neural mechanisms. *Consciousness and Cognition*, *17*(2), 523–534, figure 1, p. 527. Used with permission.)

Sensory Suppression

One of the most interesting aspects of the forward modeling/comparator account of the agentic self is that the predicted effects of planned actions typically involve suppression of the sensory consequences of predicted actions. That is, if I predict that throwing my slider at a speed of 90 miles per hour will cause a pull in my shoulder, I need not actually sense the muscle pull to model the throw and its consequences adequately (Blakemore et al., 2000). There is a sensory attenuation/suppression with voluntary but not passive motor acts. Frith (2005) has argued that delusions of control in schizophrenia are due in part to defects in the forward-modeling system that impedes the normal attenuation of sensory feedback, thereby causing patients to experience their movements as passive.

Modeling of Possible Worlds

At the core of this *comparator* model of the agentic self lies the concept of an *efference copy*, or copy of the motor command. This efference copy is actually a simulation of a possible world where the motor act actually occurs along with its sensory consequences. The whole thing therefore is an anticipatory state or better a simulation, a hallucination of a possible world that is fleeting and vanishes before the next motor act is formulated and simulated and so forth. The agentic self can use the simulation to make many valid inferences about the world, so it is a very efficient way to operate. For example, any sensory input that is not predicted from the simulation that arises from motor command would most likely come from an external event. Thus, the agent can distinguish between self-caused versus other-caused acts (i.e., agency). In addition, if the agent runs the simulation as a dynamic set of images that change in lawful ways that mimic the real world, then the agent can use the simulation to predict both sensory and other (e.g., social) consequences of the action. If the predicted consequences do not match the actual effects of the action, then the agent can tweak one parameter of the simulation at a time to see how well the possible world runs given various permutations of the basic parameters of the model. We will see below that counterfactual simulations of possible worlds are a very powerful capacity that the agentic self uses to navigate the world and to learn to optimize performance in the world.

Prospective Memory Guides Action

The agentic self uses a special memory system to maintain intentions to achieve some goal. Prospective memory (Einstein et al., 2005) keeps an intention alive until the goal is accomplished or until the goal is abandoned for one reason or another.

Prospective memory involves the retrieval of a preexisting intention, it involves remembering to remember to do something at time X (time-based prospective memory) or when a certain event occurs (event-based prospective memory). Prospective memory has a special relation to the phenomenon of temporal discounting. Temporal discounting refers to the extent to which people discount large future rewards in favor of small present rewards. Is a bird in the hand worth two in the bush? It depends on your tendency to discount future large rewards relative to present rewards. Prospective memory supports cognition about future events and rewards. The more you discount the value of future rewards, the more you are likely to find it difficult to remember to do things in the future when the time comes due. Prospective memory and reasonable temporal discounting curves makes sense only for an agentic self who has his eye on the future.

Decision Making

Perhaps the most important property of the agentic self is that it is he or she who makes the decisions about goals or choices. A number of cognitive scientists have proposed dual-processing models of decision making (Kahneman, 2003; Sloman, 1996) that involve a fast, largely unconscious and automatic system versus a slow, deliberative, reflective and conscious system. The two systems often work in tandem with each other, but sometimes they oppose each other's recommendations. When the two conflict in their recommendations, it is the reflective system that should win out when in fact the automatic system does so. To the extent that the automatic system supports habit-based and hard-wired preferences of the organism, this is probably a good thing. But when the automatic system calls the shots and overrides the agentic system's inhibition of immediate gratification of impulsive desires, trouble all too often ensues. I will have more to say about decision making in impulsivity syndromes in other chapters. Suffice it to say here that impulsivity all too often co-opts the processing resources of the automatic system, and the reflective/agentic system is often powerless to override the automatic system.

Decisions under Risk versus Uncertainty

A decision is an action, and it causes a whole series of downstream effects or resultant actions as well. Thus, decision making is a core activity of the agentic self. Decisions under risk differ from decisions made under conditions of uncertainty. Risk refers to situations where the agent knows with certainty the probabilities of possible outcomes of choice alternatives. Uncertainty refers to situations where the likelihood of different outcomes cannot be expressed with precision. In my view, many if not most uncertain situations can be reduced to risk scenarios if we assign equal probabilities to all choice alternatives that obtain in a risky scenario. If, in an uncertain situation, every outcome can occur with equal probability, then the agentic self understands with precision the riskiness of each choice he makes. What is more interesting about uncertain scenarios (now considered as scenarios bearing choice of equal riskiness) is that each choice is equally good or equally bad. So how does a rational agent choose in such a situation? If you are Buridan's ass you do nothing. Every other subcomponent of the unified self (the narrative self, the minimal self, etc.) would likely sit and do nothing when faced with two equally appealing (or unappealing) alternatives. The agentic self, however, would keep running counterfactual simulations concerning the two choices until the probabilities shifted making one choice more desirable than another (see discussion of counterfactuals later). Failing such a shift, the agentic self would choose arbitrarily because action in this case is better than inaction.

We have now completed our survey of the basic operating characteristics of the agentic self. We turn next to a consideration of how the agentic self actually works.

Models of Decision Making

Up to the modern era, most theorists assumed that agents made decisions based purely on the objective value of the thing, object, or potential outcome of the issue under consideration. But there is abundant evidence that people do not make choices based merely on the objective value of the external event or object alone. Instead, people make decisions based on some reference state or relative to some baseline state. The value of $100 to a poor man is different than its value to a rich man. The poor man is starting from a different baseline state than is the rich man. The poor man needs the money more than does the rich man. The widow's mite is worth more in the eyes of God than is the rich man's bloody sacrifice because the widow gave more than the rich man despite the vast differences in the "objective value" of the bloody sacrifice versus the widow's mite. The fact that people make decisions concerning the value of some course of action based on differing reference points is captured in various modern theories of decision making, which I review next. But note that those differing reference points at bottom simply must refer to the idiosyncratic characteristics of the agent himself. Thus, once again we see that decision making lies at the heart of the nature of the agentic self.

Counterfactual Comparisons

Perhaps the most typical way that people make decisions about competing options is via counterfactual comparisons. Counterfactual processing is therefore absolutely central to the cognitive structure that makes up the agentic self. People routinely compare the outcome of their chosen option with the outcome they could have received had they selected a closely related but different option—these are standard counterfactual comparisons. These sorts of comparisons compare an actual state of affairs, an actual world with a closely related possible state of affairs or closely related possible world. To choose intelligently among an array of options, agents construct a simulation of the world or state of affairs after a given option is chosen; call it "a." Then, agents systematically permute one or two parameters of the world model "a" and then finally run the simulation to see what would happen if these other possible worlds were chosen or made manifest.

The products of these dynamic counterfactual simulations of what might have been if things had gone slightly differently or if I had chosen option "b" instead of option "a," and so forth, can be fed into the stock of knowledge the agent uses to make decisions more generally. The products of the simulations are integrated into information stores in the cognitive system and used when necessary to make informed choices. If the integration does not occur, then the person will perhaps be less able to interpret novel experiences and thus will be less able to learn effectively from novel situations. Counterfactual processing may be crucial for this type of human learning about novelty (see papers in Byrne, 1997; Roese, 1997). Following a given outcome, particularly negative outcomes, we appraise the significance of the outcome by imagining alternatives or what might have happened if things had gone differently. We then cognitively generate simulations of imaginative scenarios that would allow or promote the alternative outcome. We do this typically by changing or mutating various causal antecedents of the outcome. We next compare the simulations of what might have been to what actually happened in an attempt to restore the unwanted outcome to a more normative routine outcome. To the extent that the comparison process reveals that the counterfactual alternatives seem plausible or possible compared with what actually happened we feel tension, distress, or discomfort and are therefore motivated to try to right the situation or to make sense of the situation. In addition, the contrastive reasoning associated with counterfactual processing may help reveal the ways in which unmet goals might be achieved (Roese, Hur, & Pennington, 1999). By engaging in these counterfactual simulations, we may more easily learn how to avoid negative outcomes in the future or we learn how to strive more effectively for current unmet goals or desired outcomes. It is as if the counterfactual mechanism activates a motivational state in us such that we strive to "make right" what had gone wrong with regard to what had almost happened.

Typically, people will tend to accept the causal implications of a counterfactual if the counterfactual is predicated on alterations of a local or specific nature rather than alterations of more general laws or universals. For example, people will more readily accept or allow themselves to learn from the causal implications of a statement like "If he had run a little faster, he would not have missed the bus" rather than from statements like "If he had been able to fly, he would not have missed the bus." Much of the research on evaluations of counterfactuals has focused on just what kinds of particular or local factors can be manipulated in *acceptable* counterfactuals. Kahneman and Miller (1986) proposed these general rules of mutability:

1. Exceptions are more mutable than routines.

2. Ideals are less mutable than non-ideals. When asked to change the outcome of a card game or tennis match, subjects do so by imagining an improvement of the losing game rather than a deterioration of the winning game.

3. Reliable knowledge is less mutable than unreliable knowledge.

4. Causes are less mutable than effects.

5. The actions of the focal or attended actor in a situation are more mutable than those of a background actor.

With these processing constraints in mind, we can see how the agentic self evaluates its past choices to make better choices in the present. The agentic self has to take these past choices seriously and allow itself to be affected by past performances such that past mistakes can be avoided. One way it does this is via emotional cognitive reactions to past mistakes.

Sometimes these emotional reactions to past mistakes take a wrong turn and become dysfunctional. Excessive rumination, for example, refers to the tendency to replay past mistakes excessively in an effort to exorcise them or to change the outcome. But typically, emotional reactions to past mistakes are functional even though painful. Regret, for example, refers to the emotion we experience when a counterfactual simulation shows how close we came to getting a past mistake or decision right. Or when regret is combined with shame it works to motivate the person to do better in the future, perhaps around moral implications of choices and behaviors. But most cases of regret are not combined with shame, and so most cases of regret are about behaviors aimed at selfish though healthy goals.

Regret Theory and the Agentic Self

The unfavorable comparison between what was received and what could have been received with a different counterfactual action is termed regret. Feelings of regret are generally more intense or stronger than feelings of triumph. Regret theory (Bell, 1982; Braun & Muermann, 2004; Loomes & Sugden, 1982) assumes that decision makers pay special attention to the emotion regret and act to avoid that emotion when making decisions of all kinds, especially financial decisions. Susceptibility to regret is a model parameter of formal regret theory and an individual difference variable that dictates the specifics of the trade-off between choice criteria. Notably, the theory depends on the assumption that people run counterfactual simulation scenarios in their minds, and as mentioned above, there is plenty of psychological and economic evidence that they do. Regret theory also makes one very special prediction that other theories do not make: People will act to minimize regret even if it means lower financial returns. In other words, people make decisions based on mental simulations about possible worlds. We will examine what happens when counterfactual simulation abilities are impaired by disease (as is the case in PD) in another chapter.

Prospect Theory and the Agentic Self

Prospect theory (PT; Kahneman & Tversky, 1979) explicitly models the decision-making process as seen from a *point of view* (i.e., from an agent who makes decisions based on the concrete situation he finds himself in). PT replaces the utility function of expected utility theory (of standard economic theory) with a value function that is defined in terms of relative gains and losses or as changes from a baseline reference point. Thus, the model is especially good at predicting what agents will do when they want to avoid loss rather than when they want to maximize gain. After all, half the battle in maximizing utility is to avoid losing what you have. But risk averseness can become too extreme and thus make risky gains impossible. A person's degree of marginal sensitivity to loss or gains at the extremes is measured by the parameter a in PTs power value function $v(x) = x^a$. Because outcomes are defined relative to a neutral reference point, the leveling off of increases in value as gains increase leads to a concave shape of the value function only in the domain of gains. This concave shape is associated with risk-averse behavior. In contrast, the leveling off of increases in disutility as losses increase leads to a convex shape of the value function in the domain of losses. This convex shape is associated with risk-seeking behaviors. Obviously, most people want to be in the middle of these two curves, but what is optimal for an agent always changes depending on the market environment and the agent's individual position in the market. Notably, risk averseness and risk seeking may be modulated to some extent by midbrain DA systems, and thus PD patients' decision making around risk will vary systematically with their levels of DA, which I will discuss in later chapters.

Summary

We have seen that the agentic self is characterized by intentionality, forethought, self-reactiveness, and self-reflectiveness. The latter two terms involve self-regulation and the former two terms capture what is essential about the agentic self: intentionality and future directedness. The agentic self formulates goals and purposes, chooses as wisely as possible among the best options via mental simulations including counterfactual comparisons, and then the agentic self pursues the goal it set for itself. Along the way, the agentic self must make adjustments, must set and meet implementation intentions, must self-monitor for progress, and must continually aim at the superordinate goal it set for itself. All these activities reduce to self-regulation. The agent uses a comparator system or prediction/error-correction system to implement intentions and to learn from mistakes and consequences of predictive simulations. Obviously, we can see some family resemblances in all of these capacities ascribed to the agentic self. Clearly, the thread that connects them all is intentionality and self-regulation toward some superordinate goal. I suggest that the agentic self's characteristic activity is best captured via the theory of self-regulation via mental simulation choice of possible selves as follows. The agentic self specializes in mentally simulating what the unified self will look like if it chooses any given option available to it. The agentic self not only chooses on the basis of potential losses and gains but also does so from a reference point, and that reference point is not the status quo per se (as PT predicts), but the reference point is some possible self the agent predicts will occur if it makes that choice. What then are possible selves?

According to Markus and Nurius (1986), possible selves are images of what people hope to become, expect to become, or fear becoming in the future. Regret theory concerns mental simulations of feared selves. PT models risk or loss aversion according to the reference point of the feared self predicted by the agentic self when it is faced with serious choices. An ideal, hoped-for self also strongly motivates people and strongly influences decision making. The ideal self is special in that it is crucial for the agentic self's efforts toward self-regulation. I will further explain the role of the ideal self later. For now I need to show how possible selves work in the process of self-regulation.

Possible selves appear to be elaborated out of imaginative mental and counterfactual simulations that obey the mutability rules laid out above. When we mentally simulate a hoped-for self, we do not allow ourselves to postulate a distantly possible world like the ability to fly, but instead we postulate a relatively closer and more realistic possible world where the self earns a higher degree or some other honor. And when we simulate feared-for selves, we do so under the mutability constraints described by Kahneman and Miller and mentioned earlier. Possible selves consist of a description of a set of behavioral actions aimed at some goal set by the agentic self along with causes and consequences of those imaginary actions, with an end state that is described as an event. According to narrative theorists (Bruner, 1995; Oatley, 2007; Ricoeur, 1984), narratives about future selves provide interpretations about what we see as possible. As stories, they help to integrate material about conflict involving the present self into a resolution of that conflict—a resolution involving a higher, more complete, and more complex self.

We evaluate our current and past selves with reference to possible selves—not the present self or the status quo (Markus & Nurius, 1986). Thus, for instance, a current representation of the self as a loss-averse individual who values future large rewards over present smaller rewards would be evaluated more severely by an individual with a salient risk-seeking possible self compared with evaluation by an individual with a "conservative" possible self. The discrepancy between the possible self as risk-seeking and the current self as loss-averse is large and has been demonstrated to be motivational. Notably, when the hoped-for self is combined with a feared possible self, the motivational strength of possible selves increases substantially because both approach and avoidance systems are activated under the regulatory control of the possible hoped-for and feared possible selves.

Possible selves become relevant for self-regulation when they are recruited into the subset of self-knowledge that is active in working memory (Markus & Kunda, 1986; Markus & Nurius, 1986). Obviously, when a possible self is periodically or chronically activated, it becomes particularly important for evaluation of current representations of the self as well as discrepancy reduction behaviors or engagement of approach and/or avoidance behaviors (Norman & Aron, 2003). For example, frequent attendance at religious services or performance of religious rituals will periodically activate a number of possible selves, including perhaps an ideal self if the person is religiously inclined. The chronically activated ideal self is then in a position to contribute to self-regulation by providing a standard by which to evaluate progress toward a goal and resolution of internal and social conflicts (Oyserman, Bybee, Terry, & Hart-Johnson, 2004).

That people use possible selves as behavioral standards to guide goal formulation and long-term self-regulation more generally has been remarked upon repeatedly (e.g., Hoyle & Sherill, 2006; Hoyle & Sowards, 1993; Kerpelman & Lamke, 1997; Oyserman et al., 2004). Hoyle and Sherill (2006) have pointed out that possible selves map particularly well into hierarchically organized control-process models of self-regulation (e.g.,; Hoyle & Sowards, 1993). Behavioral reference points or standards are organized in these models of self-regulation in a hierarchical fashion from abstract and general to concrete and specific. A particular behavioral standard derives from the level above it and so forth. The important point here is that the reference point by which agents makes choices about long-term goals is a possible self not a current self. That is why mental simulation and counterfactual comparisons are important cognitive capacities for the agentic self.

Presumably, the agentic self uses hoped-for and feared possible selves as a system for self-regulation and as a system for goal setting and realization of long-term intentions. Who do I want to become? Who do I fear becoming? These are the two mental simulations that govern the decision-making systems of the agentic self over the long term. We shall see that this regulatory scheme carries important consequences for the neuropsychiatry of PD.

4 The Neurology of the Agentic Self

Cognitive Operations of the Agentic Self

We have seen that the agentic self identifies values to be striven after, then makes decisions about which values/goals to pursue and then controls pursuit of those goals. Two important cognitive processes that contribute to a sense of agency or agentic control are decision-making processes and goal pursuit or action selection and control. I will have a lot to say about these two major components of the agentic self. But, in this chapter, I want to break down the component processes of the agentic self into a process model of how the agentic self operates (see figure 4.1). I suggest that the agentic self performs six basic serial cognitive operations that are aligned with distinctive neural systems. The agentic self (1) identifies values, (2) prioritizes them into long-term goals, (3) makes decisions about which goals to pursue, (4) develops plans to attain those goals, (5) initiates goal pursuit by inhibiting valuation and responding based on impulses alone, and (6) monitors implementation of those plans and adjusts them when necessary. In this chapter, I review what is known about the neurology of each of these basic processing operations that make up the agentic self.

The most important of these six basic operations is step 5, the inhibition of impulsive valuation and responding. All of these agentic processes require the delay of immediate gratification of impulses and the inhibition of impulsivity itself or the inhibition of the "pull" toward shorter-term salient rewards so that a longer-term perspective can be created. The agentic self must first of all have the neural power to inhibit what has traditionally been called the minimal self, which is governed by immediate rewards. In terms of neural control, the agentic self is mediated by dorsal and anterior PFC. These brain regions, when activated, inhibit activity within the ventral and orbitomedial portions of PFC as well as the belt of paralimbic

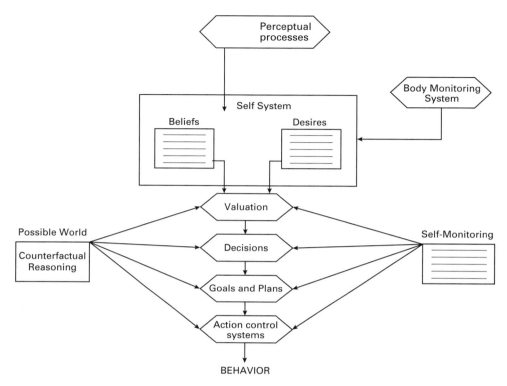

Figure 4.1
Component processes of the agentic self. (Modified from McNamara, P. 2009. *The Neuroscience of Religious Experience.* New York: Cambridge University Press.)

subcortical nuclei like the amygdala and related limbic regions. When things are running smoothly, the dorsal anterior regions exert a tonic form of control over the ventral and paralimbic cortices. In terms of dual processing network architectures, the ventral, limbic, and paralimbic regions may be thought of as supporting automatic, unconscious, stimulus-driven responding while the dorsal and anterior PFC supports reflective, conscious and more controlled, effortful, deliberative, and sometimes rational forms of decision making.

Bechara, Damasio, Tranel, and Damasio (1997) and colleagues (Burns & Bechara, 2007) have proposed a similar framework for decision making. Will power (which I subsume under the label *agentic self* or control) emerges from the dynamic interaction between an impulsive system that triggers somatic states from primary inducers and a reflective system that triggers somatic states from secondary inducers. Bechara and colleagues explicitly link their dual system architecture of will power to the two-system view of Kahneman and Tversky on *intuition* versus *reasoning* (Tversky & Kahneman, 1981). The operations of the impulsive or intuition system are fast, automatic, effortless, implicit, and habitual, whereas the operations of the reflective/reasoning system are slow, deliberate, effortful, explicit, and rule governed.

Burns and Bechara argue that these complex behaviors are the product of a cognitive process subserved by two separate, but interacting, neural systems: (1) an impulsive, amygdala-dependent, neural system for signaling the pain or pleasure of the immediate prospects of an option, and (2) a reflective, prefrontal-dependent, neural system for signaling the pain or pleasure of the future prospects of an option. The final decision is determined by the relative strengths of the pain or pleasure signals associated with immediate or future prospects. When the immediate prospect is unpleasant, but the future is more pleasant, then the positive signal of future prospects forms the basis for enduring the unpleasantness of immediate prospects. This also occurs when the future prospect is even more pleasant than the immediate one. Otherwise, the immediate prospects predominate, and decisions shift toward short-term horizons. Although during the process of weighing somatic (affective) responses the immediate and future prospects of an option may trigger numerous somatic responses that conflict with each other, the end result is that an overall positive or negative somatic state emerges. Thus, over the course of pondering a decision, positive and negative somatic markers that are strong are reinforced, whereas weak ones are eliminated. This process of elimination can be very fast. Ultimately, a winner takes all; an overall, more dominant, somatic state emerges (a "gut feeling" or "a hunch" so to speak), which then provides signals to the brain that modulate activity in neural structures involved in biasing decisions. This winner-takes-all view is consistent with the conception by Strack and Deutsch (2004) of competition between motor schemata.

Rangel, Camerer, and Montague (2008) have proposed a similar framework for conceptualizing the cognitive and neurobiologic processes that make up the decision-making capacities of an agentic self. Taking into account work from economics, psychology, neuroscience, and computer modeling, they describe a similar series of basic steps that are required for value-based decision making (Rangel et al., 2008). These basic steps are representation of the decision problem, valuation of each potential response to the problem/choice, action selection after potential responses have been rank ordered, and then an outcome evaluation process that identifies errors and makes adjustments in goal pursuit. Clearly, the only difference between my scheme and the scheme of Rangel et al. is my explicit description in step 5 of the need to inhibit impulsive responding so that more effortful forms of valuation can proceed. Rangel et al. do indeed discuss such an effortful form of valuation, but they place it under their third major form of valuation (after Pavlovian and habit), which they call goal pursuit. As far as I can see, the differences between my scheme and that of Rangel et al. is merely terminological, but I prefer my terms because I wish to emphasize effortful forms of valuation and goal pursuit as I believe these are most important for understanding neuropsychiatric disorders of PD.

For Rangel et al., representation of the decision problem might entail identifying internal states (like Damasio's somatic markers of, for example, hunger level), external states (for example, threat level) that define the problem, and then there also needs to be computation or evaluation of the pluses and minuses of various potential courses of action. To make the right decisions, the values assigned to potential courses of action have to be reliable predictors of the desired outcomes. Once an action is selected and implemented, its outcomes need to be fed-back into the decision-making process so as to make adjustments if goal pursuit has not solved the problem. Congruent with the detailed valuation and action selection process of Rangel et al., I will describe the neurology of the agentic self in terms of these sorts of decision-making and action control processes that are fundamental for any agent acting in the world.

Step 1: Identifies Values to Be Striven For

We are bombarded with all kinds of sensory impressions, stimuli, information, choices, and potential goals toward which we strive. Every agent has to sift through the welter of impressions, choices, and potential goals to strive for to identify those choices that will yield the highest value for the agent. No agent can be considered competent and truly an agent unless he can identify things of value around which to organize his actions and his goals. How is this identification of values accomplished cognitively and neurobiologically? Although it may turn out that this component process of the agentic self is not impaired in PD, we will still need to be aware of the basics of the valuation process to understand the other subcomponent processes of the agentic self. Unfortunately, little is known about the cognitive and neurobiological correlates of values identification. Rangel et al. (2008) have proposed the existence of three different types of valuation systems: Pavlovian, habitual, and goal-directed systems. These systems both facilitate and sometimes oppose one another's operations. When they conflict, the agentic self needs to enhance its executive and evaluative control processes to rank-order values and potential courses of action (see below).

The first type of valuation system proposed by Rangel et al. is the Pavlovian valuation system. It handles all the primary reinforcers that we need to live. Things like food, sex, and water are "hardwired" into our brains as values. Exposure to or attaining any of these primary reinforcers is automatically valued, particularly when we are deprived of any one of them for any length of time. The neural bases of Pavlovian valuation systems presumably involve a network that includes brain stem, periaqueductal gray, and hypothalamic drive centers as well as the basolateral and central nucleus of the amygdala, the ventral striatum, the nucleus accumbens, and the orbitofrontal cortex (OFC). These limbic and OFC sites mediate the learning processes through which neutral stimuli become predictive of the value of outcomes.

Habits imply instantiation of values chosen by the agent at some time in the past. According to Rangel et al., the habit valuation system depends on the infralimbic cortex, dopaminergic projections into the dorsolateral striatum, basal ganglia, and corticothalamic loops, which play a crucial part in learning the value of actions and turning repeated actions into habits.

Step 2: Prioritizes Values and Formulates Long-Term Goals

Rangel and colleagues' (2008) third valuation system, the goal-directed system, acts to prioritize values into long-term goals. In line with many other theorists of motor control and of agentic control more broadly speaking, Rangel et al. suggest that the goal-directed system assigns values to actions by computing action–outcome associations and then evaluating the rewards that are associated with the different projected outcomes. The computation of action–outcome associations likely depends on mental simulation abilities. For Rangel et al., the brain assigns value to simulations or *prospects* in two ways: by computing the expected rewards and risks of a potential course of action (the potential magnitude of the expected reward, its variance or coefficient of variation, and its skewness) and by computing a utility value for each potential outcome, which is then weighted by a function of the probabilities of realization of reward or nonreward. In economics, these sorts of valuation processes have been modeled by expected utility (EU) theory and by prospect theory (PT), which I discussed in the chapter on the cognitive architecture of the agentic self (chapter 3) as well as the chapter on DA (chapter 2).

In terms of neural realization of these sorts of mental simulation and decisions processes, a number of recent human functional magnetic resonance imaging (fMRI) studies have found activity that is consistent with the presence of expected value signals in the striatum and the medial OFC. In contrast, when risk is being weighed, the striatum, the insula, and the lateral OFC are activated. Underpinning both risk and expected-value signals is the midbrain DA system and its forebrain projection sites.

When mental simulations of potential courses of action return inconclusive ambiguous results and further effortful processing yields no improvements in rank ordering of potential courses of action, then the decision problem is termed *ambiguous* rather than risky, per se. When this sort of situation is prolonged, the agent adopts a harm-avoidant strategy rather than a novelty-seeking or risk-seeking strategy in its choices. This harm-avoidant personality disposition is very common among PD patients (see chapter 6 on PD personality and self) and may at least partially be due to impairment in mental simulation abilities. When simulations are impaired, then no single simulation run can be considered reliable, and thus the problem at hand is deemed ambiguous.

Consistent with the idea that mental simulations underlie the ability to assign EU and PT-derived values to potential courses of action, Rangel et al. suggest that with respect to very complex decision-making processes, individuals might use a propositional system to try to forecast the consequences of a particular action. In the language of dual system architectures alluded to earlier, the propositional system would include reflective and effortful deliberative processing that would rely primarily on dopaminergically innervated dorsal and anterior portions of the PFC. These are the systems that I am identifying most strongly with the agentic self.

Step 3: Makes Decisions about Which Goals to Pursue

Decision making is fundamental to agentic control. Formulation of goals, action selection, and long-term behavioral strategies all depend on sound decision-making processes. Decisions are made by the agent, and the neural systems that support decision making about long-term goals all converge on the specific subsystems of the PFC. The region that appears to be most important for goal choice and formulation of plans for goal pursuit and control of long-term behavioral strategies is Brodmann area 10 (BA10)—the dorsal anterior or frontopolar region of the PFC.

Notably, comparative architectonic studies of the cellular structure of BA10 (Semendeferi, Damasio, Frank, & Van Hoesen, 1997; Semendeferi, Lu, Schenker, &

Damasio, 2002; and see chapter 7 on evolutionary history of the PFC and agentic self) reveals this region to be especially complex in humans and the apes. BA10 also appears to act as a central controlling center for information flow coming from all other regions of the PFC and other association areas of the cortex. Information processing proceeds in a hierarchical fashion with BA10 as the end point in the stages of information abstraction and control. The anterior PFC is predominately (and possibly exclusively) interconnected with supramodal cortex in the PFC, anterior temporal cortex, and cingulate cortex. In addition, the number of dendritic spines per cell and the spine density are higher in BA10 than in other comparable areas of the cortex, but the density of cell bodies is markedly lower. This indicates that a lot of computational work and integration of information occurs here.

As just summarized, BA10 is at the end of a processing hierarchy, and thus it is integrative with respect to the information that flows into it from other regions in the hierarchy. Its output is to other supramodal regions of the cortex and very likely includes actual decisions made, intentions to act, and selection of actions and goals to implement intentions. Thus, executive control over both the processing of information and of actions occurs only via this BA10-anchored processing hierarchy. The processing hierarchy respects and reflects the anatomic organization of the PFC, whereby posterior and caudal frontal regions support control involving temporally proximate, concrete action representations, and the rostral and anterior PFC supports control involving temporally extended, abstract representations. As cognitive content "moves" from posterior to anterior sites or from top to bottom regions, information or action commands become much less abstract and general and much more concrete and specific. Every action command is represented hierarchically and sequentially. For example, to make a sandwich you first must decide which sandwich to make and then gather the ingredients, and this gathering is represented under a node called "making a sandwich." Under the node "gathering the ingredients," you must create a further branching of nodes like "open the fridge," "take out the mustard and cold-cuts," and so forth. Thus, control of even the simplest of actions requires commands that are hierarchically specified in terms of superordinate goals and subgoals and concrete motor outputs.

There are several theories of hierarchical executive control systems in the PFC, and they are all relevant to an understanding of the ways in which an agentic self might operate. Fuster's (2004, 2008) perception–action cycle proposes that as actions are specified from abstract plans to concrete responses, progressively posterior regions of lateral frontal cortex are responsible for integrating more concrete information over more proximate time intervals. Burgess, Gilbert, and Dumontheil (2007) propose that BA10 operates as a kind of biasing mechanism or gateway that coordinates the relative amounts of stimulus-dependent, externally oriented versus stimulus-independent, internally oriented forms of thought that support goal pursuit. Christoff and Gabrieli (2000) (a similar scheme is proposed by Ramnani & Owen, 2004) suggest that the PFC and the anterior region in particular handles progressively more relationally complex forms of information. As we proceed in a rostro-caudal gradient in the frontal lobe, more and more complex forms of relational information can be held in working memory. First-order relational complexity (e.g., "what is the color?") is associated with ventrolateral prefrontal cortex (VLPFC). Second-order relational complexity (e.g., "do the colors match?") is associated with DLPFC. Third-order relational complexity is associated with BA10 and entails evaluation of relationships among relationships.

The model of PFC function that I think best captures the data relevant for agentic control processes is the so-called "cascade model" (see figure 4.2) proposed by Koechlin and Summerfield (2007) (a similar model was proposed by Badre & D'Esposito, 2007). Koechlin and Summerfield suggest that agentic control involves selection of pieces of information derived from internal and external sources (contextual information) that can act as control signals for ongoing actions/goal pursuit. As I read the model, control signals are selected from among alternative action representations that are constructed out of contextual information matched to internal intentional states. As we progress along the PFC anatomic hierarchy, greater levels of control are made possible. The control signal developed in a previous level is used to construct a new control signal that embodies what was controlled in the previous level and adds to it more contextual information at the next level of control and therefore more control. Separate signals are processed by spatially distinct regions along the rostro-caudal axis of the PFC. Some actions only require a sensory stimulus to be emitted and to work. Sensory control is supported by premotor cortex. Next, the posterior PFC selects an action based on proximate environmental contextual cues (contextual control). Anterior DLPFC supports episodic control, which in turn will use contextual and sensory control signals to output episodic actions. Finally, at the highest level, *branching control*, supported by BA10, selects action representations based on a *pending*, or prospective, temporal context. Thus, from caudal to rostral regions of the PFC we get greater and greater distance from control by the immediate sensory context. In BA10, we get the greatest distance from immediate sensory control of actions, and instead prospective future-oriented actions are the norm. In support of the cascade model, Koechlin et al. performed neuroimaging of brain activity while volunteers selected one of two

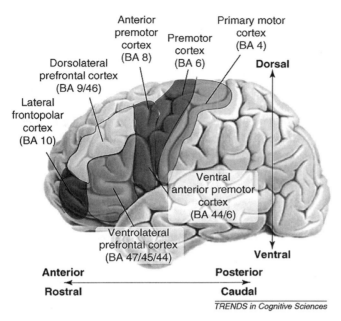

Figure 4.2
Schematic of major anatomic subdivisions in the frontal lobes. Boundaries and Brodmann areas (BAs) are only approximate. Arrows indicate anatomic directions of anterior/rostral (front) versus posterior/ caudal (back) and dorsal (up) versus ventral (down). From caudal to rostral, labeled areas include motor cortex, dorsal (PMd) and ventral premotor cortex, dorsal (pre-PMd) and ventral aspects of anterior premotor cortex, VLPFC and DLPFC, and lateral frontal polar cortex (FPC). (From Badre, D. 2008. Cognitive control, hierarchy, and the rostro-caudal organization of the frontal lobes. *Trends in Cognitive Sciences*, *12*(5), 193–200. Used with permission.)

button-press responses based on cues that varied along three dimensions depending on closeness to sensory control/context. The dorsal premotor cortex was active across all three levels, the anterior premotor/posterior DLPFC was active across sensory and context levels, and the anterior DLPFC was active only for the highest episodic level.

Step 4: Develops Plans to Attain Those Goals

One of the most robust neuropsychological paradigms that assesses development of plans is the Tower of London (TOL) task. In a typical version of this task, three beads—one blue, one red, and one yellow—have to be moved from a starting configuration on three sticks of unequal length to a target arrangement in a minimum number of moves. Subjects are asked to rearrange the beads on the sticks so that their positions match those of the target array (presented as a colored drawing). The starting position of the beads is varied so that in any particular trial, the solution can only be reached after a minimum of 2, 3, 4, 5, or 6 moves. The respondent's task is to solve the problem with the minimum number of possible moves. Each subject is given four trials of each problem with 2, 3, 4, 5, or 6 moves. The number of problems solved correctly with the minimum number of moves is the outcome score. Neuroimaging studies have demonstrated DLPFC activation in subjects attempting to solve the problem. Lange et al. (1992) reported improved performance on the TOL in patients with PD after administration of the dopaminergic drug LD.

Step 5: Initiates Goal Pursuit by Inhibiting Impulses Associated with the Minimal Self

I have claimed above that step 5 is the most important for operation of the agentic self. In order for the agent to identify values, rank order them, choose among them, and implement goal pursuit based on those choices, the impulsive self needs to be inhibited and controlled by the reflective or agentic self. I propose that when the reflective self inhibits the minimal/impulsive self, the individual feels a sense of agency or will power. How does the reflective/agentic self inhibit the impulsive self?

When people report this feeling of agency or will power, a widely distributed network of brain regions are activated including premotor cortex (ventral PMC), the SMA, the DLPFC, the posterior parietal cortex (PPC), the posterior segment of the superior temporal sulcus (pSTS), and the insula (Blakemore, Frith, & Wolpert, 2001; Farrer & Frith, 2002; Farrer et al., 2003; Fink et al., 1999; Jeannerod, 2004; Leube et al., 2003). Notably, these are regions that receive connections from BA10.

All the major nodes in this widely distributed network are known to send inhibitory efferents onto target structures along the ventral axis coursing from the limbic system up to the ventromedial PFC. This limbic and ventromedial PFC system supports what has traditionally been called the minimal self. Literally hundreds of studies have demonstrated that people preferentially remember words that (they think) refer to themselves (e.g., curious) versus words that they deem refer to another person. This preference for words referring to the self is known as the *self-reference effect* (Symons & Johnson, 1997). When participants perform these sorts of self-reference tasks (deciding if an adjective describes them or another, etc.), the medial prefrontal cortex (mPFC) virtually always becomes activated. In addition, this region is implicated in autobiographical memory and impulsivity.

The minimal self may overlap considerably with what has become known as the *default network* of brain sites that sustain basic levels of activation even when the subject sits and does nothing but daydreams. Just as the reflective system is hypothesized to suppress activation levels in the impulsive minimal self system, so, too, goal-directed thought reliably suppresses default network activity. In my terms, activation of the agentic self network reliably suppresses activity within the default network sites that overlap with minimal self network sites.

One of the primary benefits of suppression of the impulsive minimal self is the ability to delay gratification of impulses in favor of longer-term goals and larger rewards. People differ in their propensity to discount larger future rewards in favor of smaller short-term rewards. The extent to which people can avoid this propensity to discount future rewards is a measure of the strength of the agentic self. Discounting or inappropriate devaluation of large future rewards results from the dominance of the minimal self over the agentic self. The minimal self operates with a high discount rate and the reflective self with a low discount rate. Consistent with the gateway hypothesis concerning the function of BA10, it may be that BA10 integrates computations performed by limbic and ventral PFC regions (within the minimal self) regarding immediate outcomes (stimulus-dependent thought) with computations performed within the striatal-dorsolateral PFC (within the agentic self) regarding delayed outcomes.

Step 6: Monitors and Adjusts

If the agentic self is going to improve in its control procedures and in its choices, it needs to learn from its mistakes. For learning to happen, the system must monitor events that are "off-track," events that represent less than the expected reward. When something happens that does not meet the predictions derived from the choices, plans, and goals created by the agentic self, then that unexpected event has to be recorded and fed back into the system so that it can be used to make better predictions in the future. Every time a less than expected reward occurs, that information is used to update prediction computations to make them more accurate. The comparison of what was predicted with what actually occurred can be modeled in so-called "feed-forward comparator models."

Summary of the Operations of the Agentic Self

To sum up results of the discussion presented in this chapter: The agentic self (1) identifies values, (2) prioritizes them into long-term goals, (3) makes decisions about which goals to pursue, (4) develops plans to attain those goals, (5) initiates goal pursuit by inhibiting valuation and responding based on impulses alone, and (6) monitors implementation of those plans and adjusts them when necessary.

The most important of these six basic operations is step 5, the inhibition of impulsive valuation and responding. This boils down to suppression of the minimal self by activation of the agentic self. The agentic self is mediated by dorsal and anterior PFC with BA10 acting as the key node in the network mediating executive control processes. These brain regions, when activated, inhibit activity within the ventral and orbitomedial portions of PFC as well as the belt of paralimbic subcortical nuclei like the amygdala and related limbic regions. When things are running smoothly, the dorsal anterior regions exert a tonic form of control over the ventral and paralimbic cortices. The temporal discounting curves differ for the two selves. The minimal self processes information about short-term rewards, whereas the agentic self processes information about larger long-term rewards. BA10 may integrate these two discounting biases. In terms of dual processing network architectures, the ventral, limbic, and paralimbic regions may be thought of as supporting automatic, unconscious, intuitive, stimulus-driven responding, and the dorsal and anterior PFC supports reflective, stimulus-independent forms of thought as well as conscious and more controlled, effortful, deliberative, and rational forms of decision making. In normal functioning, the two systems operate in a kind of mutual inhibitory balance but with a strong tonic bias in favor of the reflective system. When the minimal self gains the upper hand for a long period of time (of the order months), the individual becomes vulnerable to all kinds of pathology. If the agentic system is not able to inhibit portions of the amygdala that mediate fear or negative affect, for example, then the individual may become vulnerable to anxiety or depression. If the agentic self is not able to inhibit rewards pathways within the minimal self system, then the individual may become vulnerable to impulsive responding and so forth. In the chapters that follow, we will see examples of these sorts of breakdown patterns in the PD population.

5 Impairment of the Agentic Self in Parkinson's Disease: Cognitive Deficits in Parkinson's Disease

In previous chapters, I have defined the nature and functions of the agentic self. In this chapter, I will show that selective cognitive subcomponents of the agentic self are impaired in PD and that this information helps us to understand both the normal cognitive operations of the agentic self and the symptomatology and functional impairments associated with several of the neuropsychiatric disorders of PD.

Neuropsychiatric Disorders of PD as Impairments of Subcomponents of the Agentic Self

I suggest that many of the symptoms of the psychiatric disorders seen in some PD patients can best be explained as impairments in the agentic self. That is, these patients are best described as suffering impairments in the agentic self rather than as suffering impairments in executive functions or in decision making, and so forth. Why attempt to understand neuropsychiatric symptoms as breakdowns in the functioning of the self rather than as isolated impairments in various cognitive processes like decision making or executive cognitive functioning? For one thing, characterizing the mental dysfunction of PD as an impairment in the agentic self helps to unify most, if not all, mood and cognitive problems of PD. We will see that beyond the consistently reported ECF and mood impairment in PD, there is, for example, a specific language-related deficit in speech act production and comprehension. Speech acts express the agentic self accomplishing some act with language. To say "I promise . . ." is to perform the act of committing oneself (one's agentic self) to a course of action vis-à-vis some other person. The profile of premorbid (increased anxiousness and harm-avoidance behaviors; decreased novelty seeking) and post-onset personality changes of PD are also consistent with an impairment in agentic self. I will discuss other mood and cognitive problems of PD later, and it will be seen that they all can be usefully understood as impairments in an agentic self system.

In addition, cognitive processes are impossible to understand fully without invoking their functions. Given that most cognitive processes function in service to the self, it seems reasonable to attempt to understand deficits in these cognitive processes as linked with an overarching deficit in the self. Attentional capacity and focus, for example, varies according to the desires, beliefs, and values of the self. Attentional dysfunction, therefore, will either be caused by or influence functioning in the self system. Decisions are made by the self in the interests of the self and to further the goals of the self. Breakdowns in the decision-making process will, therefore, either be caused by or influence the functioning of the self system. Planning is done in service to goals formulated by the self. Breakdowns in planning will be influenced by breakdowns in the self system. Memory exists to provide the self with a fund of information on past mistakes and triumphs so that it can learn to avoid mistakes and to repeat triumphs. If the self system is impaired, memory processing will inevitably be affected. Language exists to communicate intentions, ideas, desires, emotions, and acts of the self. If the self system breaks down, all agentic aspects of the language faculty will be affected. Rationality itself probably evolved to develop strategic aims of the self in its competition with others and with the adversity of the natural world. If the self system is impaired, rational choice processes will be altered in a way that reflects the impairments in the self system.

Cognitive processes are also very often linked-up into chains of operations that follow one upon another. You cannot fully understand a cognitive process without identifying its place in the processing chain and the ultimate function of that chain of cognitive processors. The ultimate function of a chain of cognitive processing systems is to advance the strategic aims of the self system. It is standardly argued, for example, that in the normal course of events, a perceptual stimulus hits the retina, is sent to visual centers in the brain where its primitive features are analyzed and packaged together into an object, and this object representation is then sent to other parts of the brain that then attach meaning to the "object." But, this standard picture is false as it leaves out the self. From start to finish, it is important to realize that information pickup is not neutral and that once information is picked up, it is not processed in a neutral manner. Instead, the stimulus is processed in such a way as to be of maximum service to the agent. The agent decides what is noticed and then perceived. A real live human being does not scan the environment like some unbiased photographic machine picking up everything it sees. If it did so, it would rapidly get overloaded with information and then crash. Instead, a real human being *selectively* scans the environments looking *selectively* for rewards or threats; he preferentially opts for perceptual pickup of emotionally relevant stimuli . . . he chooses to see a predator in the shadows instead of mere shadows, even though objectively speaking all that is out there is shadow.

Once a decision is made concerning the predator in the shadows, the information is "sent" downstream to inform and guide action (i.e., production of plans to meet the threat). The information is not processed in some neutral or objectively efficient manner. The brain at this stage does not try to produce an unbiased report of the raw data in as efficient a manner as possible. Instead, the information is shunted rapidly into agentic control centers that can rapidly recruit metabolic and mental resources to eliminate or kill the predator. Plans are rapidly formulated to defend against the predator and potentially to harm or kill the predator. These plans, in turn, are translated into motor programs that implement the plans and so forth. It is only after all this automatic processing takes place that the reflective system can kick in and gather further perceptual information concerning the threat to see if it remains, is real, or if it was not a threat or is no longer a threat. Thus, information processing occurs in a serial manner with one processing system using the products of the previous processing system to make decisions that it then sends downstream to the next processor, and so on. If one link in the chain is impaired, it affects all downstream links in predictable fashion. When we adopt the perspective of the agentic self, we automatically construe cognitive processes as strategic operations biased to serve the interests of the agent, and we automatically see processing systems as linked in a chain of such systems that serve the interests of the self. Instead of examining cognitive deficits in isolation, we can examine effects of a deficit on other processing systems in the chain that affects the self.

Cognitive processes operate as links in a chain that facilitate the strategic aims of the agent or self. To understand those cognitive operations, we need to see how they work in concert with other cognitive processes to serve the interests of the agent. When we take that strategic perspective, the perspective of the agentic self, we are better able to identify consequences of cognitive breakdown for psychiatric disorders. If, for example, we find that a PD patient with depression has an impairment in the cognitive process we call *planning*, we can identify the deficit and leave it at that. But, that would be mere description and slavish empiricism. If, instead, we look at where in the series of cognitive processing systems "planning" comes in, we can identify downstream consequences of the planning deficit. If, for example, planning comes after decision making but before goal identification and motor programming, then motor output should be reduced, and attainment of long-term rewards should be reduced. If an individual fails to plan for long-term rewards, he will never obtain those rewards, and if he fails to attain long-term rewards, this will have consequences for his depression.

No cognitive operations are neutral with respect to the goals and the aims of the self. If we leave out the self, we risk losing the big picture. Of course, it is perfectly reasonable to study the functioning of various cognitive systems without referring them to the self. But, eventually, to really understand the role, the powers, the nature, the capacity, and the constraints of each cognitive system we study, we need to refer them back to the strategic aims of the self. This research strategy is nothing more than to advocate that the study of cognitive disorders should adopt the Darwinian perspective. Within the evolutionary framework, animals, including human beings, are treated as strategic agents who work to further their long-term genetic and reproductive interests. There can be no physiologic system that is not strategic in this sense. Every individual animal and, therefore, every individual human being is a strategic agent. Its physiologic systems, including its cognitive systems, function strategically to further their genetic interests in the reproductive contest. At the human level, this means that talk of an agentic self will be useful.

Against Deflationary Accounts of the Self

In human beings, the strategic behavioral orientation is captured in what we call the self (more specifically the agentic self). There are many theoretical accounts of the self (see the review in Boyer et al., 2005). Deflationary accounts of the self claim that it is empty, that there is no little man sitting up there in the brain making decisions and formulating plans, and so forth. Of course, there is no homunculus in the brain making decisions, but there is a physical location in the brain where some kind of final "decision" is made. It is false to say that there is no agentic structure or process that can be properly called the self. There is an abundance of cognitive and psychological data that demonstrate beyond any doubt that a self system exists, it uses resources, and it exerts real effects in the world (see, for example, the papers in Baumeister & Vohs, 2004). The self system can be characterized in many different ways such as a set of abstract schemas or procedural rules or memory images, or narrative structures or mental simulations or verbal scripts, and so forth (see papers in Sedikides & Spencer, 2007). No matter how one characterizes the representational medium of the self, the fact remains that there is such a system and that system (or at least specific "selves" that I have been calling the minimal self and the agentic self) is instantiated in the brain in relatively specific neural networks (see papers in Feinberg & Keenan, 2005). The representational system and its associated neural networks have special properties relative to other cognitive structures. The agentic self system has unique and privileged access to all kinds of internal information (like visceral feeling and pain) and it controls pickup of all kinds of external information. Most importantly, the self system (or at least its agentic arm) controls behavioral output of the individual and does so (via specification of goals) over the entire lifetime of the individual. No other cognitive system has these special properties or powers. Thus, we are licensed to speak about the agentic self as a specific entity, process, or system in the brain just as we do any other cognitive system. It has measurable properties that emerge from and transcend the cognitive processes that subserve its operations and that are controlled by it. Its structure can be revealed by its breakdown patterns like any other complex cognitive system. To say as do some of the deflationary theorists concerning the self that the self is nothing but the set of primitive cognitive operations that mediate its operations is at best a trivial observation, and more accurately, a non sequitur. In a trivial sense, the self system like all other complex cognitive systems draws on more basic cognitive operations to perform its operations. But, this tells us nothing interesting about the self system, per se. To understand the nature and power of language, for example, it is not that interesting to point solely to a more primitive set of cognitive operations that support language expression. *All* complex mental functions are composed of more primitive operations. Surely, the interesting thing about language (and the self system) is to see how combinations of various primitive operations produce uniquely powerful mental capacities and talents. The language faculty produces all kinds of absolutely new cognitive products and whole cultures. It cannot be accurately captured via an enumeration of basic cognitive operations that support its operations. Of course, it is equally beside the point to ignore the basic subcomponents of a complex system. To do so would result in ignorance of its fundamental operating characteristics. We obviously need to aim at understanding the basic components of a complex system without succumbing to the mistake that these basic subcomponents are all that the system is. To do justice to complex systems, it is necessary to keep in mind and attempt to characterize the unique emergent properties of these systems as well.

It is an error to assume that a complex mental operation is nothing but its supporting operations. Every complex mental structure or operation when it has shown that it can persist over time despite interference transcends the primitive operations that gave rise to it. In short, new things emerge from old things, and when they do so emerge they are actually real things with properties that are not entirely reducible to the old things. The things or properties that are not reducible to the old things are precisely those properties that appear when the new things emerge from the old things. You cannot get those properties without the new emerging from the old. Only the new thing displays those properties. With respect to the self, it surely does emerge from more primal cognitive processes such as the executive functions, language, memory, somesthesis, and so forth. But, once the self emerges from these more basic processes, it displays properties and capacities that are unique to the self system and that cannot be found in any of the aforementioned basic processes. Without the self system, these new special properties would never appear, nor would the basic subsystems be seen operating in tandem with one another. With respect to the self system, the new emergent properties include all of the self-related emotions like shame, pride, envy, regret, and the like. They include the axiological aspects of cognition such as valuation, prospection, purpose, desire, instrumental rationality, and so forth. They include certain structural features of language such as the agent slot in argument structures and in thematic roles, the subject–object grammatical structure of many languages, the first-person personal pronoun complex and related anaphora, speech act verbs, and so forth. They include that fundamental aspect of self-consciousness we call reflexivity or the ability to reflect upon oneself. Even *intentionality*, or that capacity to direct the mind toward some object in the world, is dramatically reshaped by the appearance of the reflexive capacities of the self. No longer is intentionality controlled merely by the object of its gaze, but with the capacity for reflexivity we can make the self itself the object of intentions and thus a "project." In short, the self is real, it exhibits complex cognitive structure, it uses mental and metabolic resources, it has effects in the world, and we ignore it at our peril.

I now return to an examination of the agentic self in PD.

Control of Agentic Self over Operations of the Minimal Self

I suggest (see figure 4.1) that the agentic self performs six basic serial cognitive operations that are aligned with distinctive neural systems. The agentic self (1) identifies values, (2) prioritizes them into long-term goals, (3) makes decisions about which goals to pursue, (4) develops plans to attain those goals, (5) initiates goal pursuit by inhibiting the minimal self, and (6) monitors implementation of those plans and adjusts them when necessary. I will be suggesting that step 5 (inhibition of the *minimal self*) is the major problem in PD but that step 3 (decision making) is also altered very early in PD. Thus, the PD patient has no problem identifying values and rank ordering them in terms of appropriateness and importance. The patient's decision-making process, however, is skewed in terms of greater harm avoidance than is necessary. His ability to develop plans is unimpaired, but when it comes time to initiate goal pursuit, he cannot muster enough inhibitory force to suppress operations of the minimal self, and thus, mental simulation processes (which require the agentic self to be in control of the minimal self) are weak, and downstream processes of monitoring and control are impaired. In short, the agentic self is weak in PD (likely due to reduced activation in PFC networks from ascending mesocortical DA afferents) and is never able to control the minimal self fully and is never able to implement its agenda fully.

In terms of neural control, we have seen that the agentic self is mediated by dorsal and anterior PFC. These brain regions, when activated, inhibit activity within the ventral and orbitomedial portions of PFC as well as the belt of paralimbic subcortical nuclei like the amygdala and related limbic regions. The latter set of regions mediates expression of the minimal self. In terms of dual processing network architectures, the ventral, limbic, and paralimbic regions may be thought of as supporting automatic, unconscious, stimulus-driven responding, and the dorsal and anterior PFC supports reflective, conscious and more controlled, effortful, deliberative, and sometimes rational forms of decision making. If the agentic self is never able to suppress operations of the minimal self effectively, then reflective, controlled, effortful cognitive processes like the ECFs and mental simulation processes (like counterfactual processing and decision making) will be impaired.

In what follows, I will evaluate the extent to which each of the six major cognitive processes of the agentic system are intact or impaired in PD. I begin with a summary review of the evidence concerning regional brain dysfunction in PD. If the agentic self is selectively impaired in PD, then we would expect greater dysfunction in the dorsolateral and anterior PFC and related networks rather than in the midline paralimbic, ventromedial, and orbitofrontal cortices.

Brain Dysfunction in PD

Is the agentic neural system impaired in PD? First of all, it is clear that most patients with PD exhibit impairments in the ECFs that have been linked with both dorsolateral and the anterior PFC as well as the anterior cingulate cortex and some parietal networks (see review below in the section "Step 5: Initiates Goal Pursuit"). In addition, non-PD patients with lesions to the DLPFC usually exhibit impairments in sustained attention, working memory, and/or set maintenance and shifting in response to changing task demands—the same set of impairments typically seen in many midstage PD patients. Thus, the neuropsychological data appear to support the view that the agentic self system is selectively impaired in PD. What about direct measurement of brain function in PD? Is the network that supports the agentic system impaired in PD?

Recently, a new technique has been used to look at networks rather than isolated brain regions in various neurologic disorders. Specifically, spatial covariance analysis (Hirano, Eckert, Flanagan, & Eidelberg, 2009) has been successfully used to identify network abnormalities that are associated with neurodegenerative diseases including PD, Alzheimer's disease (AD), and Huntington's disease (HD). This technique applies principal components analysis to data obtained from neuroimaging scans and identifies metabolic covariance patterns related to disease. It turns out that the PD-related spatial covariance pattern (PDRP) is characterized by *increased* pallidothalamic and pontine activity (likely linked with motor deficits), which covary with relative metabolic *reductions* in the premotor cortex, SMA, DLPFC, and parieto-occipital association regions (likely linked with both motor and cognitive deficits in PD). To date, the PDRP has been identified in seven different patient populations scanned in the rest state with either fluorodeoxyglucose (FDG) PET or ECD SPECT perfusion imaging.

An even more specific network pattern has been linked with cognitive and affective changes in PD. This PD-related cognitive pattern (PDCP) is correlated with impairments in memory and executive functioning and is characterized by reduced metabolic activity in prefrontal and parietal cortices, with relative increases in dentate nuclei and cerebellar hemispheres. Thus, results from attempts to identify impairments in neural networks in PD (via application of the spatial covariance analysis) implicate the agentic DLPFC in cognitive and affective deficits of early PD.

There are also studies of the extent of cerebral atrophy in the brains of living PD patients. In a very carefully conducted recent study (Burton, McKeith, Burn, Williams, & O'Brien, 2004), the pattern of cerebral atrophy on magnetic resonance imaging (MRI) in PD patients with and without dementia was established. The investigators used voxel-based morphometry (VBM) to provide an unbiased means of investigating brain volume loss. Whole-brain structural T1-weighted MRI scans from PD patients with dementia (PDD; $n = 26$), PD patients without dementia ($n = 31$), AD patients ($n = 28$), patients with dementia with Lewy bodies (DLB; $n = 17$) and control subjects (n = 36) were acquired. Images were analyzed using SPM99 and the optimized method of VBM. We are interested in results in the patients without dementia. PD patients without dementia showed reduced gray matter volume in the frontal lobe compared with that of control subjects. The investigators concluded that PD without dementia involves gray matter loss in frontal areas apparently including dorsal PFC. When patients become demented in late stages of the disease, the atrophy extends to temporal, occipital, and subcortical areas. Thus, these data on cerebral atrophy in PD are consistent with the idea that the PFC is the site of impairment in early and mid stages of the disease. The DLPFC is the key "node" in the network I have been claiming as mediating the agentic self. In summary, results from neuropsychological and neuroimaging data support the view that the DLPFC is impaired even in early PD.

I next present evidence for impairment in PD for several of the steps, or cognitive processes, that are constitutive of the agentic self's operations. We will see that the evidence for impairment exists for steps 3–6 but that identification of values to be striven for and the ability to rank order those values appears not to be impaired in PD.

Step 1: Identifies Values to Be Striven For

Every agent has to sift through the welter of impressions, choices, and potential goals to strive for to identify those choices that will yield the highest value for the agent. No agent can be considered competent and truly an agent unless he can identify things of value around which to organize his actions and his goals. As far as I can tell, this component process of the agentic self is not impaired in PD. Patients with PD are able to express consistently what they desire, value, and need.

Step 2: Prioritizes Values

When an individual identifies values or the things that are important to him, he typically also ranks them in order of preference or importance. Patients with PD appear to have little problem prioritizing their goals and values. We (McNamara, Durso, & Harris, 2006) compared the priorities assigned to various life goals in a group of patients with PD and age-matched controls. Patients with PD produced consistently lower mean importance ratings on all the life-goals measured in the study. Patients with PD were less likely than age-matched elderly controls to cite religion, social contacts, leisure activities, and personal care as "extremely important life goals." Persons with PD assigned significantly lower "importance" ratings to leisure activities and religion than did controls. The goals rated most important by persons with PD were family, residential arrangements, and the relationship with partner. These priorities are similar to the control group and are congruent in terms of life priorities (with the exception of the lower rating on religion) with what has been found in larger population studies.

Step 3: Makes Decisions

Decision making is fundamental to agentic control. Formulation of goals, action selection, and long-term behavioral strategies all depend on sound decision-making processes. Decision-making processes, in turn, depend on more fundamental abilities to produce and run mental simulations in one's mind. When making a decision that requires any amount of thought, we try to imagine what might be the outcome or consequences associated with choosing y over x and so forth. We construct imaginary scenarios of what might happen when we make a choice after weighing all the options. When the ability to construct and run mental simulations is impaired, then no single simulation run can be considered reliable, and thus the problem at hand is deemed ambiguous, and poor decisions are made. Can patients with PD construct and run effective mental simulations of potential alternative outcomes or courses of action? The available data suggest that the answer is no. Consider the case of counterfactual processing abilities of PD patients.

Counterfactual Processing in PD   Counterfactuals are mental simulations of "what might have been" or "what might be" if x is chosen over y. They refer to imagined alternatives to something that has actually occurred or to something that might happen once a decision is made. They play a significant role in other cognitive processes such as conceptual learning, decision making, social cognition, mood adjustment, and performance improvement (Roese, 1999). They help us to process causal relations by highlighting possible causal antecedents of an unpleasant outcome (e.g., "if only we had left earlier, we would have avoided the storm," "if I choose x over y, I will risk only a small loss") and to imagine better ways of proceeding ("Henceforth, we will leave earlier . . ."; ". . . study harder . . ." ". . . take fewer risks . . .," etc.). Without counterfactual thinking, a person would find it more difficult to avoid repetition of past mistakes, to adjust his or her mood after an unpleasant event, to reason effectively about unpleasant events, and so forth.

We (McNamara, Durso, Brown, & Lynch, 2003) administered tests of counterfactual generation and counterfactual reasoning to a group of patients with PD and control participants. We found that patients with PD were significantly less likely to generate counterfactual thoughts after recalling a negative memory and in response to direct questions than were control participants. Controls produced double the number of counterfactuals as that produced by the PD patients. In addition, scores

Table 5.1
The Counterfactual Inference Test (Hooker et al., 2000)

---

1. Janet is attacked by a mugger only 10 feet from her house. Susan is attacked by a mugger a mile from her house. Who is more upset by the mugging?
(a) Janet (20.0; 40.0; 86.0)
(b) Susan (6.7; 0.0; 0.0)
(c) Same/can't tell (73.3; 60.0; 14.0)

2. Ann gets sick after eating at a restaurant she often visits. Sarah gets sick after eating at a restaurant she has never visited before. Who regrets their choice of restaurant more?
(a) Ann (46.7; 10.0; 7.0)
(b) Sarah (40.0; 50.0; 88.0)
(c) Same/can't tell (13.3; 40.0; 5.0)

3. Jack misses his train by 5 minutes. Ed misses his train by more than an hour. Who spends more time thinking about the missed train?
(a) Ed (40.0; 10.0; 7.0)
(b) Jack (40.0; 70.0; 91.0)
(c) Same/can't tell (20.0; 20.0; 2.0)

4. John gets into a car accident while driving on his usual way home. Bob gets into a car accident while trying a new way home. Who thinks more about how his accident could have been avoided?
(a) Bob (53.3; 40.0; 88.0)
(b) John (26.7; 20.0; 5.0)
(c) Same/can't tell (20.0; 40.0; 7.0)

Note: Correct or normative responses to these questions are (1) a, (2) b, (3) b, (4) a. Numbers in parentheses represent percentage (%) of PD patients who selected this item ("percentage of undergraduates" in Hooker et al. pilot validating study).
Source: From McNamara, P., Durso, R., Brown, A., & Lynch, A. (2003). Counterfactual cognitive deficit in patients with Parkinson's disease. *Journal of Neurology, Neurosurgery, and Psychiatry, 74,* 1065–1070. Used with permission.

on the Counterfactual Inference Test (CIT; Hooker, Roese, & Park, 2000) were significantly higher for controls compared with those for patients with PD. The PD CIT scores were approximately what would be expected if the test options were selected at random. It can be seen from table 5.1 (see the percentage response selections in parentheses) that PD patients selected their answers in a distinctly atypical pattern relative to the normative responses of healthy people. Items 1 and 3 reflect the fact that counterfactual thinking is enhanced for events that nearly happened over that for events that did not (item 1 is spatial, item 3 is temporal), whereas items 2 and 4 focus on the fact that counterfactual thinking is typically enhanced for unusual rather than normal events. PD patients performed atypically on all items but were most atypical for the "nearly happened" items (items 1 and 3) and those requiring evaluation of affective responses (items 1 and 2: "Who is more upset . . ."; "Who regrets . . . more . . ."). For example, whereas 86% of the normative sample selected "Janet" as the person who would be most upset, presumably because she was only 10 feet from safety when the mugging occurred (the "nearly happened" response), only 19% of PD patients did so. Seventy-one percent of the PD group selected the "don't know–can't tell" response for the same item. Similarly, only 28.5% and 38% of PD patients selected the normative responses for items 2 and 3, respectively. PD patients approximated the normative response only for question 4—a question requiring a judgment of "who thinks more about how to prevent a future accident." These results indicate that impairment both in counterfactual thinking and in counterfactual-derived inferences are associated with PD.

PD Patients and the Iowa Gambling Task   One of the neuropsychological tests specifically developed to evaluate decision-making processes in brain-injured populations is the Iowa Gambling Task (IGT; Bechara, Damasio, Damasio, & Anderson, 1994). This task has been administered to patients with PD and thus has yielded valuable information concerning decision-making processes in PD. In the IGT, subjects are given four decks of cards and $2,000 in play money with which to play a game. The goal is to win as much money as possible. Subjects repeatedly choose cards from the four decks. On the back of each card, the subject is told how much money he wins or loses. Decks A and B are associated with high gains but also occasionally very high losses. These are the disadvantageous decks. If the individual persists in drawing cards from these decks, his overall earnings will decline rapidly. Decks C and D are advantageous, drawing lower rewards per card, but also incurring smaller penalties such that playing mostly from these decks leads to an overall gain.

Healthy subjects very quickly learn which decks will lead to better outcomes (usually by about card 80). In this task, risks (the cards in the disadvantageous decks) are obviously associated with losses, whereas in the real world people are rewarded for taking risks. Nevertheless, the task is an ingenious and reliable method for assessing people's willingness to incur risk despite being punished with losses.

Poletti et al. (2010) have examined several studies of decision-making deficits in PD (Brand et al., 2004; Czernecki et al., 2002; Delazer et al., 2009; Euteneuer et al., 2009; Ibarretxe-Bilbao et al., 2009; Kobayakawa, Koyama, Mumura, & Kawamura, 2008; Mimura, Oeda, & Kawamura, 2006; Pagonabarraga et al., 2007; Perretta, Pari, & Beninger, 2005; Thiel et al., 2003).with several of these papers relying on the IGT to measure decision making. The general trend of the findings from all these papers suggests that PD patients perform as well as control subjects on some outcome measures of the IGT but have difficulty learning to avoid losses and in fact are either insensitive to punishment (loss) or actually prefer risky choices. Two papers (Czernecki et al., 2002; Euteneuer et al., 2009), however, reported findings that at first seem inconsistent with these general conclusions concerning PD decision-making deficits.

The Euteneuer et al. (2009) study is particularly interesting as the authors attempted to directly compare two forms of decision making: decisions taken under ambiguity and decisions taken under risk. The investigators pointed out that the IGT assesses decision making under ambiguity whereas another game, the Game of Dice Task (GDT), assesses decision making under risk. People with lesions in the limbic–orbitofrontal–striatal loop, the neural network I have argued that supports the minimal self, typically do poorly on the IGT but not the GDT, which has been associated with the DLPFC–striatal loop. I have linked the DLPFC–striatal loop, or network, with the agentic self. People with lesions in the DLPFC–striatal loop do poorly on the GDT. Euteneuer et al. (2009) studied performance of 21 nondemented PD patients on both tasks. The patients were tested while they were on dopaminergic medication. The authors found that PD patients were significantly impaired in the GDT but not in the IGT. Performance on the GDT was correlated with measures of ECF. In both tasks, PD patients showed significantly reduced feedback electrodermal responses (EDRs) after losses, but not after gains, indicating a primary decline of sensitivity to negative feedback. Tasks (the GDT and the executive function tasks) that require activation of the DLPFC (the agentic self in my terms) were performed particularly poorly. The authors concluded that the primary problem was dysfunction in the DLPFC–striatal loop. But, if the problem is in the DLPFC–striatal loop, why the reduced EDR sensitivity to negative feedback (losses)? The authors themselves suggest that reduced EDRs were due to dysfunction in the limbic loop. But, then, why didn't the PD patients perform poorly on the IGT as well, which the authors themselves argued was dependent on the limbic–orbitofrontal (OF) loop? I suggest that poor activation in the DLPFC loop enhances dysfunction/dysregulation (overreactivity) in the limbic loop. The limbic–OF loop is overactive (patients were tested while on dopaminergic medications) because the DLPFC is underactive. Reduced sensitivity to negative feedback but relatively preserved performance on IGT is due to hyperactive limbic–OF loop, whereas poor performance on GDT is due to reduced activation in the DLPFC. All of these decision-making data are therefore consistent with the idea that the agentic self as mediated by the DLPFC–striatal loop is impaired in PD and is causally linked with both decision-making deficits and limbic dysfunction.

Step 4: Develops Plans to Attain Those Goals

One of the most robust neuropsychological paradigms that assesses development of plans is the Tower of London (TOL; Shallice, 1982) task. PD patients exhibit consistent deficits on this task even in the early stages of the disease (Culbertson, Moberg, Duda, Stern, & Weintraub, 2004; Morris et al., 1988; Owen, 2004; Owen et al., 1992; Taylor & Saint-Cyr, 1995; Taylor, Saint-Cyr, & Lang, 1986), but it appears that the PD deficit only emerges when patients are confronted with less predictable subgoal sequence planning. The easy version of the planning task can be done by PD patients, but when complexity increases, even with the addition of a single subgoal sequence, PD performance declines. In a typical version of the TOL task, three beads—one blue, one red, and one yellow—have to be moved from a starting configuration on three sticks of unequal length to a target arrangement in a minimum number of moves. Subjects are asked to rearrange the beads on the sticks so that the positions of the beads match those of the target array (presented as a colored drawing). The starting position of the beads is varied so that in any particular trial, the solution can only be reached after a minimum of 2, 3, 4, 5, or 6 moves or subgoals. The respondent's task is to solve the problem with the minimum number of possible moves. Each subject is given four trials of each problem with 2, 3, 4, 5, or 6 moves. The number of problems solved correctly with the minimum number of moves is the typical outcome score. The available data suggest that the TOL task depends primarily on striatal–prefrontal networks (Owen, 2004). Lange et al. (1992) reported improved performance by PD patients on the TOL after administration of the dopaminergic drug LD.

Step 5: Initiates Goal Pursuit

I have claimed above that step 5 is the most important for operation of the agentic self. In order for the agent to identify values, rank order them, choose among them, and implement goal pursuit based on those choices, the impulsive self needs to be inhibited and controlled by the reflective or agentic self. I propose that when the reflective agentic self inhibits the minimal/impulsive self, the individual feels a sense of agency or will power. How does the reflective/agentic self inhibit the impulsive self in order to initiate goal pursuit?

The Feeling of Agency   When people report this feeling of agency, a widely distributed network of brain regions is activated including the ventral premotor cortex (vPMC), the SMA, the DLPFC, the PPC, the pSTS, the insula, and the cerebellum (Blakemore, Frith, & Wolpert, 2001; Farrer & Frith, 2002; Farrer et al., 2003; Fink et al., 1999; Jeannerod, 2004; Leube et al., 2003). Note that all of these areas are the same regions implicated in the cascade theory of PFC with the addition of the PPC, the pSTS, and the insula. Notably, these are regions that also receive connections from BA10. In short, the feeling of agency is strongly associated with activation in the network of structures we have identified with subserving the agentic self.

PD Temporal Discounting   One of the primary benefits of suppression of the impulsive minimal self is the ability to delay gratification of impulses in favor of longer-term goals and larger rewards. People differ in their propensity to discount larger future rewards in favor of smaller short-term rewards. The extent to which people can avoid this propensity to discount future rewards is a measure of the strength of the agentic self. If the agentic self is impaired in PD, then we would expect a tendency to discount heavily future large rewards in favor of short-term smaller rewards. The critical factor appears to be the level of DA activity in the striatum. Enhancing DA activity in the striatum to above normal levels increases impulsivity by enhancing the reward value of immediate rewards over future rewards (temporal discounting) (Pine, Shiner, Seymour, & Dolan, 2010). Impulsivity syndromes in PD patients who have been given dopaminergic agonists has been well documented. Decreasing DA activity to below normal levels in PD patients likely also leads to inability to value accurately future rewards relative to immediate rewards, but as of this writing (December 2010), I know of no published studies on temporal discounting in PD.

Impairment in Frontal/Executive Cognitive Functions   Activation of the agentic self normally inhibits the networks associated with the minimal self, but in PD, the agentic self is impaired. This is evidenced by the suite of deficits that have been documented in the area of ECFs in PD. As mentioned previously, PD patients have been shown, for example, to exhibit impairments in working memory, planning, response monitoring, set shifting, and attentional control. PD patients are also known to perform poorly on the standard neuropsychological tests that are thought to measure executive function such as the Stroop Color-Word Interference Test, the Wisconsin Card Sort Test (WCST), and verbal fluency tasks. Gotham et al. (1988) and Lange et al. (1992) reported improved fluency performance (relative to the off state) after LD administration in PD patients indicating that these tasks depended in part on adequate DA levels in the system. In a typical verbal fluency task, subjects are instructed to produce as many items (words) as possible for each category (the letter *F* or *A* or *S* or the category *animals*) within 60 seconds.

In the alternating condition, subjects are asked to alternate between letter and category generation. For each fluency test, the number of correct words (i.e., total words minus repetitions and proper names) and number of correct alternations per minute are tallied; the greater the number of responses, the better the performance. In the WCST, the subject is required to sort response cards according to one of four stimulus conditions as defined by the designs on the cards. After 10 consecutive correct sorts, the examiner shifts the required sorting principle to one of the other stimulus dimensions. The subject has to discover, through trial and error and examiner feedback, what the new sorting principle is. Although the WCST should not be considered a selective "frontal" test, regional cerebral blood flow (rCBF) studies show that DLPFC networks are activated during the card sorting task (Weinberger, Berman, & Zec, 1986). Kulisevsky et al. (1996) reported improved performance of PD patients on the WCST at optimal drug levels but poor performance at nonoptimal levels. Similarly, Gotham et al. (1988) report impaired performance on WCST in the on state, but this, as the authors suggested, may have represented excessive dopaminergic stimulation in the PFC in the patients they tested. The Stroop (1935) procedure requires the subject to name the color of the ink in which a color-word is printed. Sometimes the word will name the color of the ink (the word *blue* in blue ink), and sometimes the word will be the name of a different color than the ink (e.g., the incongruent word *blue* printed in green ink). The subject must ignore the word and name the color. Susceptibility to cognitive interference is calculated as a ratio of the time taken to name the colors in the incongruent condition compared with the time taken to read the words in the congruent condition (*interference cost*).

Step 6: Monitors and Adjusts

When something happens that does not meet the predictions derived from the choices, plans, and goals created by the agentic self, then that unexpected event has to be recorded and fed back into the system so that it can be used to make better predictions in the future. One of the breakthroughs in cognitive neuroscience in the past decade has been the finding that phasic bursting of midbrain DA neurons encodes and sends a prediction-error signal to sites in the limbic system and in the PFC when unexpected outcomes occur. Every time a less than expected reward occurs, that information encoded in the phasic signal is used to update prediction computations to make them more accurate. The comparison of what was predicted with what actually occurred can be modeled in so-called feed-forward comparator models, which I covered in chapter 3.

Prospective Memory Deficits in PD

To monitor implementation of plans and goals, people use what has been called *prospective memory*, or remembering to carry out previously formed intentions or plans (McDaniel & Einstein, 2007). Successful prospective memory requires several executive control processes that depend on the DLPFC and anterior PFC network that I have identified with the agentic self. To remember to do something in the future, the individual presumably has to plan to do something at a particular moment in the future, maintain that intention until the time arrives to implement the plan, and then perform the intention or plan when the time or event arrives that calls for the "plan." All of these prospective control capacities are capacities that the agentic self has to be able to perform to carry out executive control tasks. The available data suggest that PD patients are impaired in event-based prospective memory tasks and perhaps even in time-based prospective memory tasks, though the data here are less clear (Altgassen, Zöllig, Kopp, Mackinlay, & Kliegel, 2007; Katai, Maruyama, Hashimoto, & Ikeda, 2003; Kliegel, Phillips, Lemke, & Kopp, 2005). The impairment in event-based prospective memory in PD patients cannot be attributed to loss of information in memory concerning the original plan or intention. When given cues to elicit that information, PD patients readily produce the requisite information and successfully perform the prospective task. This suggests that individuals with PD have intact encoding and storage of the intention (consistent with steps 1 and 2 described earlier) but are unable to output the intention/plan at the appropriate moment. This is an agentic impairment. PD patients also perform poorly with respect to everyday prospective memory tasks in real-life contexts. They forget to take their medications at the appropriate time or forget to make calls or keep appointments and so forth.

Notably, prospective memory appears to be especially dependent on activation in anterior or frontopolar PFC BA10 (Burgess, Scott, & Frith, 2003). This region, as I suggested in the chapter on the neurology of the agentic self (chapter 4), is a key node in the neural network that supports agentic executive control of behavior.

Summary

To sum up results of the discussion presented in this chapter: The agentic self (1) identifies values, (2) prioritizes them into long-term goals, (3) makes decisions about which goals to pursue, (4) develops plans to attain those goals, (5) initiates goal pursuit by inhibiting the minimal self (valuation and responding based on impulses alone), and (6) monitors implementation of those plans and adjusts them when necessary. PD patients are impaired in steps 3–6. They have difficulty making decisions, developing plans, inhibiting the minimal, impulsive self, and monitoring and adjusting plans and actions.

The most important of these six basic operations is step 5, the inhibition of automatic or impulsive valuation and responding in order to initiate goal pursuit. This boils down to suppression of the minimal self by activation of the agentic self. I presented neuroimaging, physiologic, and behavioral evidence that suggests that the neural network that supports operations associated with the agentic self is impaired in PD. Pathologic and behavioral evidence points to dysfunction in DLPFC and the frontopolar cortex in PD. The agentic self is mediated by dorsal and anterior PFC with BA10 acting as the key node in the network mediating executive control processes. These brain regions, when activated, inhibit activity within the ventral and orbitomedial portions of prefrontal cortex as well as the belt of paralimbic subcortical nuclei like the amygdala and related limbic regions. In PD, the diminution in phasic bursting of DA neurons leads to weak or ineffective activation in the neural networks that support the agentic self, and the result is ECF deficits, deficits in mental simulation, in prospective memory, planning, discounting of future rewards, and so forth.

In terms of dual processing network architectures, the ventral, limbic, and paralimbic regions may be thought of as supporting automatic, unconscious, intuitive, stimulus-driven responding, and the dorsal and anterior PFC supports reflective, stimulus-independent forms of thought as well as conscious and more controlled, effortful, deliberative, and rational forms of decision making. In normal functioning, the two systems operate in a kind of mutual inhibitory balance but with a strong tonic bias in favor of the reflective agentic self-system regulating the impulsive, automatic minimal self. When (due to a weak agentic self) the minimal self gains the upper hand for a long period of time (of the order months), the individual becomes vulnerable to all kinds of pathology. I will show in the following chapters that in the extreme case of PD (with dramatic loss of dopaminergic activity in the agentic system), the weak agentic self system/hyperactive minimal self system contributes to the symptomatology of the neuropsychiatric syndromes we see in PD. For example, the agentic system is not able to inhibit portions of the amygdala that mediate fear or negative affect, so the individual may become vulnerable to anxiety or depression. If the agentic self is not able to inhibit reward pathways within the minimal self system, then the individual may become vulnerable to impulsive responding and so forth.

I have been arguing that PD is characterized by weak activation of the neural networks, the striatal–DLPFC/frontopolar cortex, that support the agentic self, the self that identifies, values, formulates plans, makes decisions, initiates actions, and acts. Because the dorsal prefrontal systems normally regulate and inhibit ventral, OF, and limbic systems, the weak activation in striatal/prefrontal circuits in turn leads to hyperactivity in various limbic, amygdalar, and OF circuits. The combination of dorsal prefrontal hypoactivation and ventral prefrontal/limbic hyperactivation contributes to all the neuropsychiatric disorders of PD. In addition, the system imbalances also lead to some characteristic personality traits of PD. These characteristic traits contribute to neuropsychiatric symptomatology as well, so it will be necessary to review them in some detail. The characteristic personality alterations of PD are expected under the theory I have been presenting here. A weak agentic self system and a resultant hyperactive amygdalar and limbic/OF system should yield a personality profile of low novelty seeking (due to weak agency), high harm avoidance, depressive affect, and high anxiety levels (due to hyperactivity in amygdalar circuits).

One of the fascinating things about personality characteristics of PD is that there is fairly good evidence that the personality can be recognized decades before the onset of the motor symptoms of PD. This evidence for a premorbid personality of PD as well as similar findings with respect to depressive and anxious affect appearing decades before the motor problems appear suggest that the illness really begins in forebrain centers rather than in the brain stem or rather that forebrain centers are implicated along with brain-stem pathology right from the beginning of the disease process. Whatever the merits of this conjecture, there is now no question but that there are certain personality traits that are characteristic of someone with parkinsonism. It will be my claim that these personality traits are due to the weak activation of the agentic self system. I turn now to a review of the evidence for all these claims.

Evidence for a Premorbid Personality in PD

Eatough, Kempster, Stern, and Lees (1990) studied personality profiles of young-onset patients with PD. They found that these patients were more cautious, less flexible, more conventional, and stereotyped in thought. Hubble and Koller (1995) studied 35 PD patients and 35 controls with a personality inventory. The investigators asked the spouses of the PD patients to complete the adapted personality inventory on the personalities of their spouses for the period 5 years prior to disease onset and then for the current period. The control spouses completed the personality period for 10 years prior and currently. PD patients were found to be "less talkative" and "flexible" and more "generous," "even-tempered," and "cautious" before the onset of their motor symptoms. The results of Mendelsohn, Dakof, and Skaff's (1995) (based on patient and caregiver recollections of premorbid personality traits) are also consistent with the claim of an introverted premorbid personality type. Glosser et al. (1995) asked relatives of 29 patients with PD to complete the extensive personality inventory, the NEO ("neuroticism," "extraversion," and "openness to experience"; the NEO also measures "agreeableness" and "conscientiousness"), on the patients for the period when patients were in their thirties and for the current period. They also asked a group of relatives of patients with AD to do this task as well. Whereas there was evidence for a premorbid personality type among both patient groups, the premorbid traits were very similar so the authors argued against a distinctive premorbid PD personality. Bower et al. (2010) collated data on 6,822 healthy subjects who were followed over four decades as part of a longitudinal Mayo Clinic study on personality and aging. All of these participants had been given a version of the Minnesota Multiphasic Personality Inventory (MMPI) at the beginning of the study. Two hundred twenty-seven of these subjects developed parkinsonism (156 developed PD). When the authors assessed the extent to which baseline MMPI scores were related to PD onset, it was found that an anxious personality profile was associated with an increased risk of PD [hazard ratio (HR), 1.63; 95% confidence interval (CI), 1.16–2.27]. A pessimistic personality trait was also associated with an increased risk of PD but only in men. A depressive profile was *not* related to PD onset. When anxiety, pessimism, and depressiveness were combined into a single neuroticism scale, this scale, too, predicted later parkinsonism. Notably, significant effects were obtained for this scale even when the

MMPI was administered early in life many decades earlier (with subjects aged 20–39 years old). Thus, the personality profile that best predicted PD onset *some five decades later* was an "anxious" and "neurotic" profile that was obtained when these people were young adults. Several case-control or cohort studies (reviewed in Savica, Rocca, & Ahlskog, 2010) have suggested that anxiety may be one of the earliest manifestations of PD even when analyses are restricted to 20 or more years before PD onset. In summary, anxiety and neuroticism may predate motor symptoms of PD by more than 20 years. This personality profile may, therefore, be one of the earliest biomarkers for the disease currently known. REM sleep behavior disorder (RBD) can precede PD onset, but typically, it does not appear until 5 or 10 years before onset. The same is true with other potential clinical biomarkers such as constipation. Thus, the premorbid personality of PD may be the earliest clinical biomarker for risk of the disease that we have.

This latter result raises the issue of whether genetics plays a role in creating a vulnerability to both an anxious personality style and ultimate PD. Twin studies might be able to shed some light on this question, but I could identify only three such studies. Duvoisin, Eldridge, Williams, Nutt, and Calne (1981) studied 12 monozygotic twin pairs discordant for PD. The affected twins were found to be more nervous and introverted than their twins. Ward et al. (1984) studied 20 twin pairs discordant for PD and found (based on retrospective recall by them and their relatives) that the affected twin at age 8 was less usually the leader and more self-controlled; 10 years before onset of PD, the affected twin was still less usually the leader, more nervous, and less adventurous than the other twin. Heberlein, Ludin, Scholz, and Vieregge (1998) studied 15 German-speaking twin pairs discordant for PD; 6 monozygotic (MZ) twin pairs (4 men); 9 dizygotic (DZ) twin pairs (5 men); and a group of controls. Twins with PD scored lower than controls and their twin counterparts in "achievement orientation" and "extraversion," and they scored higher in "inhibitedness," "somatic complaints," and "emotionality."

The PD Personality Persists Through the Course of the Illness
Many clinicians who specialize in PD have suggested that PD may be associated with a specific social style or personality type—a personality profile that cannot be due merely to reactions to chronic disease. Notably, this personality type is consistent with the premorbid personality profile ascribed to PD patients. This *parkinsonian personality* has been described as socially withdrawn, rigid, punctilious, serious, stoic, introverted, and uninterested in others. The first controlled study of personality features of PD that I could find in the English language literature was by Booth

(1948). Before the late 1940s, the literature on nonmotor and personality symptoms of PD was largely anecdotal and observational. In addition, these observations of patients with the shaking palsy may have included all kinds of variants of parkinsonian-type disorders rather than the disorder we call PD today. Despite the uncontrolled nature of the observations made of people with parkinsonism, it is a remarkable fact that certain trends emerge in these clinical observations (table 6.1). The psychoanalysts tended to note that the patients had a weak ego but were deeply aggressive in their dreams; the non-Freudian psychiatrists pointed to the high intelligence, rigid moralism, and industriousness of many of their patients, and the neurologists tended to find similar traits in their patients.

Booth (1948) used clinical interviews and the Rorschach method to study personality changes in 66 patients with various types of parkinsonism and a group of patients with arterial hypertension as controls. He also claimed to have examined handwriting specimens of 16 patients produced before the onset of parkinsonism, but he quotes another author for the source of these data. In any case, Booth claimed that the parkinsonian personality is characterized by an urge toward action, expressed through motor activity (thus, the tremor) and through industriousness; striving for independence, authority, and success within a rigid, usually moralistic, behavior pattern. Booth also noted that many of his patients suffered from marked claustrophobia—an anxiety disorder. We will see that anxiety disorders are a constant of PD both premorbidly and throughout the course of the disease.

Prichard, Schwab, and Tillmann (1951) examined 100 patients with various forms of parkinsonism and concluded that their personalities fell into one of the following groups: group A (48 patients) were stable, easy-going personalities; group B (33 patients) were suggestible and dependent personalities; and group C (19 patients) were driving, restless, and assertive. He argued that these differing personality types responded differentially to medical treatments with groups A and B responding favorably to most medications and only 37% of group C responding favorably to treatment. This observation of Prichard and colleagues (1951) that patients with a distinct personality profile (group C) has not been adequately followed up. Prichard and his colleagues were later to claim a fourth group of PD patients existed that evidenced frank psychopathology.

Machover (1957) studied the responses to Rorschach figures of 42 patients with various form of parkinsonism. He argued that personality changes depended on duration of the disease and so he compared responses of patients who had the disease for a short period with patients who had the disease for a long period of time. Across both groups, he claimed to have found evidence for cognitive interference, dependence, affective instability, inertia, and passivity. The groups differed in the amount of constriction, rigidity, and inertia they expressed in their responses with greater amounts of these responses occurring in the long-duration group.

Our research team has also documented alterations in the PD self and personality relative to both healthy age-matched controls and to other patients with chronic neurologic impairments such as low back pain, aphasia, AD, and cardiovascular disease (McNamara & Durso, 2000, 2003; McNamara, Durso, & Brown, 2003; McNamara, Durso, & Harris, 2006, 2007; McNamara, McLaren, & Durso, 2007; McNamara, Obler, Au, Durso, & Albert, 1992). Using a sentence stem-completion task that allows one to classify respondents into one of several personality profiles, we (McNamara et al., 2003) found that whereas 12.84% of PD responses were classified as "impulsive/self-protective," only 7.5% of age-matched control responses were so classified. The bulk of PD responses were classified as "socially conformist" (36%) or transitional between "conformism" and "conscientious" (28%). The corresponding percentages for controls were 41% "conformist" and 32% "transitional." A conformist social style implies a reduced investment in a more independent and autonomous style. This reduction in autonomy, of course, should not be surprising in a progressive disorder like PD. Analysis of PD responses as a function of Hoehn–Yahr disease stage revealed that patients classified into stage 3 produced a greater percentage (an increase of 14%) of conformity responses compared with that of stage 2 patients and, conversely, fewer "conscientious" responses (decrease of 16%) than that of stage 2 patients, suggesting a shift toward a conformist sense of self as the disease progresses. Paradoxically, while the disease promotes a greater and greater reliance on others, it simultaneously undermines the ability of the patient to understand the motives and intentions of others. This latter problem may then lead to an overall inclination to withdraw from others.

A number of studies of the self and personality in PD have investigated the tendency to withdraw from interactions with others. A number of these studies have used Cloninger's (1987) Tri-dimensional Personality Questionnaire (TPQ) to assess three dimensions of personality that characterize various styles of social actions and interaction. These fundamental aspects of the agentic self are called *novelty seeking* (NS), *harm avoidance* (HA), and *reward dependence*. Most of these studies have documented reduced novelty-seeking responses and high harm-avoidance profiles in PD patients (Kaasinen et al., 2001; Mathias, 2003; McNamara, Durso, & Harris, 2007; McNamara, McLaren, & Durso, 2007; Menza, Golbe, Cody, & Forman, 1993;

Table 6.1

A summary of previous research examining personality in PD divided into premorbid, current, and twin studies

Author and Date	Location	Population Studied	Mean Age ± SD, Years (Range)	Mean PD Duration, Years (Range)	Mean Hoehn–Yahr Stage (Range)	Medication Information	Control Group Studied
Premorbid Personality							
Booth, 1948	USA and Germany	66 mixed parkinsonism patients including encephalitic parkinsonism (46 males)					Patients with arterial hypertension
Eatough et al., 1990	England	Young-onset PD patients (number of each sex not given)	46.1 (no range)	9.7 (no range)	Not given	Not given	25 patients with rheumatoid arthritis and 28 normal subjects
Menza et al., 1990	New Brunswick, NJ	20 PD patients (8 males)	61.8 (no range)	6.5 (no range)	2.1 (no range)	13 PD patients taking carbidopa/LD; 7 PD patients taking selegiline (Deprenyl) and were receiving no dopaminergic drugs	Spouses, close family friend, and 20 controls (8 males)
Poewe et al., 1990	Austria and Germany	38 PD patients (22 males)	54.9 (44–77)	5.2 (1–11)	2.7 (2–4)	All but 1 on LD therapy mean duration 4.2 years (5–17 years); mean daily dose 610 mg (300–1,200 mg)	20 patients with essential tremor (11 males) and 17 healthy individuals (11 males)

Matching Criteria	Mean Age ± SD, Years (Range)	Mean Disease Duration for Control Group, Years (range)	Personality Measure(s) Used	Overall Findings
			Rorschach method and in 16 cases analysis of the graphic characteristics of handwriting specimens produced before the onset of parkinsonism	The parkinsonian personality is characterized by urge toward action, expressed through motor activity and through industriousness; striving for independence, authority, and success within a rigid, usually moralistic, behavior pattern. 3. The following factors appear to be responsible for this personality structure: (a) Constitutional, probably hereditary emphasis on aggressiveness, functional prevalence of the locomotor function, tendency toward identification with a dominant parent figure, responsiveness to social values. (b) The accident of an inferior position regarding competition in childhood, perhaps also a low general vitality. 4. The disease symptoms appear when the personality attitude cannot be carried on successfully. They satisfy the dominant needs of the parkinsonian on a symbolic level: compulsive activity of the motor system and rigidity of behavior. Goal-directed actions are restricted to emotionally accepted purposes and must appear likely to be successful. Aggression is also expressed through increased salivation.
Age, sex, and occupational status	47.2 (no range); age not given for normal individuals	15.8 (no range)	California Psychological Inventory (CPI) and the Eysenck Personality Questionnaire (EPQ)	PD patients were more cautious, less flexible, more conventional, and stereotyped in thought.
Age and degree of disability	61.6 (no range)	11.2 (no range)	Tridimensional Personality Questionnaire (TPQ); PD patients and controls completed the TPQ based on the present and how they were 20 years ago; spouses and a close friend of the PD patients completed the TPQ based on how the patient was 20 years earlier.	PD patients exhibited less novelty seeking than controls. Patients rated the TPQ similar to spouses and family friends.
Age and sex	Essential tremor: 65.6 (54–77) Healthy individuals: 59 (no range)	Not given	Cattell's 16 PF personality inventory; subjects also were administered a semistructured interview to assess premorbid characteristics.	No clear differences between PD patients and those with essential tremor; patients were found to be more socially alert, apprehensive, tense, driven, etc.

Table 6.1
(continued)

Author and Date	Location	Population Studied	Mean Age ± SD, Years (Range)	Mean PD Duration, Years (Range)	Mean Hoehn–Yahr Stage (Range)	Medication Information	Control Group Studied
Premorbid Personality							
Hubble et al., 1993	Leavenworth, KS	35 PD patients (26 males)	61 ± 4.2 (no range)	5.8 ± 3.1 (no range)	1.9 ± 5 (no range)	Not given; inclusion criteria mention responsiveness to LD	35 controls (26 males)
Glosser et al., 1995	Philadelphia, PA	29 PD patients (20 males)	PD patients: 66 ± 8.9 (no range)	PD patients: 10.3 ± 7.2 (no range)	PD patients: 2.3 (1–3)	Not given	13 AD patients (7 males), 13 medical controls (4 males) with rheumatoid arthritis and osteoporosis. A close relative of each patient.
Mendelsohn et al., 1995	California	41 PD patients (23 males)	50–80	10	80% were stage 3–4	Study reports that all but one were taking the standard medications prescribed for PD; no medications for PD listed	38 spouses of PD patients, 48 married couples from a community sample (48 males); 1/3 reported a chronic medical condition
Bower et al., 2010	New York	6,822 healthy subjects were followed over four decades; 227 of these subjects developed parkinsonism (156 developed PD)					

Matching Criteria	Mean Age ± SD, Years (Range)	Mean Disease Duration for Control Group, Years (range)	Personality Measure(s) Used	Overall Findings
Age and sex	Not given	Not given	Adapted Personality Inventory (PI) from Brooks and McKinlay (1983); PD spouses completed the PI 5 years prior to disease onset and currently for patients; control spouses completed the PI for 10 years prior and currently.	PD patients were found to be "less talkative" and "flexible" and more "generous," "even-tempered," and "cautious" before the onset of their motor symptoms. The PD patients seemed to have changed more since the onset of the disease.
Age, education, occupation, or disability	AD patients: 76.2 ± 5.9 (no range) Medical controls: 63.7 ± 5.8 (no range) Close relative: NA	AD patients: 3.6 ± 1.8 (no range) Medical controls: 10.5 ± 8.1 (no range) Close relative: NA	NEO-PI: Ratings were obtained on the NEO-PI for how the patient (or control) is currently and how the patient (or control) was in his or her thirties (premorbid). Relatives, PD patients, and medical controls completed the ratings twice.	Evidence for the premorbid syndrome was supported but the profile is not distinctive as PD patients were rated similarly as AD patients.
Age, community, religious affiliation, number of years married	Spouses: Not given Community sample: Not given	Spouses: Not given Community sample: Not given	Adjective Checklist (ACL); self-administered to patients, spouses, and married couples: patient-now, patient-before, spouse-now, spouse-before	Patients and their spouses had similar ratings on the ACL. They both agreed on what traits had changed among patients.
			Minnesota Multiphasic Personality Inventory (MMPI)	An anxious personality was associated with an increased risk of PD (HR, 1.63; 95% CI, 1.16–2.27). A pessimistic personality trait was also associated with an increased risk of PD but only in men.

Table 6.1
(continued)

Author and Date	Location	Population Studied	Mean Age ± SD, Years (Range)	Mean PD Duration, Years (Range)	Mean Hoehn–Yahr Stage (Range)	Medication Information	Control Group Studied
Current Personality							
Prichard et al., 1951	Boston, MA	100 parkinsonian patients					
Machover, 1957	New York City	42 parkinsonian patients	Patients split into 2 groups with short vs. long duration of PD: mean ages are 52.8 for group I and 46.4 for group II	6 months to 38 years			
Jiménez-Jiménez et al., 1992	Spain	33 PD patients (16 males)	Males: 69.6 ± 1.95 (no range) Females: 70.1 ± 1.64 (no range)	Not given	Males: 2.87 ± 0.26 (no range) Females: 2.65 ± 0.27 (no range)	5 PD patients untreated; 28 PD patients treated with anti-parkinsonian drugs alone or in combination including LD (28 cases), bromocriptine (19 cases), amantadine (2 cases), and anti-cholinergics (3 cases)	66 controls (32 males)
Menza et al., 1993	New Brunswick, NJ	50 PD patients (sex not given)	63.8 (no range)	7.7 (no range)	2.3 (no range)	Mean LD dose 495 mg; no other medication info given	31 medical controls (rheumatology or orthopedic illnesses)
Menza et al., 1995	New Brunswick, NJ, and London, UK	9 PD patients with bilateral PD (5 males); they also had a twin*	Mean age is not given; age range is 47–78; mean age is 65	6 (no range)	2.3 (no range)	Patients were tested off anti-parkinsonian drugs, which were stopped 12 hours before scan; mean levodopa dose 480 mg	No control group

Matching Criteria	Mean Age ± SD, Years (Range)	Mean Disease Duration for Control Group, Years (range)	Personality Measure(s) Used	Overall Findings
			Clinical interviews; 12 were given Rorschach, and 15 were given a Cattell personality inventory	Patients were divided into the following personality types: A (48 patients), normal stable, easy-going personalities; B (33 patients), suggestible and dependent personalities; C (19 patients), driving, restless, and assertive personalities. Both groups A and B responded favorably to medical therapy, (79% and 77%), whereas only 37% of group C responded favorably.
			Rorschach protocols	The Rorschach patterns of 30 PD patients yield no evidence of a consistent personality picture with emphasis on an aggressive drive toward activity, independence, and mastery, which is in conflict with fear of failure and a high level of social-minded morality. Rather, the data point more to cognitive interference, dependence, affective instability, inertia, and passivity. The Rorschach differences between the short duration altered in the direction of constriction, rigidity, and inertia.
Age, sex, and cultural level	Males: 69.1 ± 1.83 (no range) Females: 69.8 ± 2.23 (no range)	NA	Spanish version of the MMPI	Female PD patients obtained higher scores on the following scales: hypochondria, depression, hysteria, and social introversion.
Age and degree of disability	64.1 (no range)	10.1 (no range)	TPQ	PD patients had less novelty seeking than controls.
NA	NA	NA	TPQ	PD patients underwent [18F]fluorodopa PET, and the trait novelty seeking was found to correlate with less uptake of DA in the left caudate.

Table 6.1
(continued)

Author and Date	Location	Population Studied	Mean Age ± SD, Years (Range)	Mean PD Duration, Years (Range)	Mean Hoehn–Yahr Stage (Range)	Medication Information	Control Group Studied
Current Personality							
Fujii et al., 2000	Kanto area of Japan	67 PD patients (29 males)	64.12 ± 9.23 (no range)	Not given	2.90 ± 0.57 (range 1–4)	31.4% of the sample was taking antidepressant drugs; no PD medications given	69 healthy, unrelated controls (36 males)
Jacobs et al., 2001	Germany	122 young-onset PD patients (71 males)	44.9 ± 4 (33–50)	8.1 ± 6.4 (1–34)	2.3 ± 0.9 (no range)	Mean dose of LD 394 ± 232 mg	122 healthy controls (71 males)
Kaasinen et al., 2001	Turku, Finland	Part I: 61 (41 males) unmedicated PD patients Part II: 47 (33 males) unmedicated PD patients	Part I: 62.1 ± 7.9 (47–79) Part II: 62.7 ± 7.7 (47–79)	Part I: 5 (no range) Part II: not given	Part I: NA; 31.9 ± 7.4 (14–53). Part II: not given	Patients were tested without drug; paper states that no patients had received any anti-parkinsonian drugs or any other medications that would influence dopaminergic neurotransmission	Part I: 45 healthy controls (19 males) Part II: NA
Tomer & Aharon-Peretz, 2004	Haifa, Israel	40 PD patients (28 males) divided according to side of disease onset. Left-onset: 18 (13 males) Right-onset: 22 (15 males)	Left-onset: 66.7 ± 9.1 (no range) Right-onset: 62.7 ± 9.0 (no range)	Left-onset: 3.7 ± 2.9 (no range) Right-onset: 4.1 ± 4.1 (no range)	Left-onset: 1.5 ± 0.67 (no range) Right-onset: 1.5 ± 0.8 (no range)	Left-onset: 3 patients unmedicated; 10 on LD; 2 on dopaminergic agonists; 7 on MAO inhibitors; 3 on anticholinergics. Right-onset: 3 patients unmedicated; 13 on LD; 5 on DA agonists; 7 on MAO inhibitors; 2 on anticholinergics.	17 healthy controls (8 males)
McNamara et al., 2008	Boston, MA	34 PD patients (33 males)	70.6 ± 11.1 (no range)	Not given	2.6 ± 0.69 (no range)	Only mentions that patients were tested while on some form of dopaminergic medication	17 controls (10 males) with chronic disease (e.g., low-back chronic pain syndromes)

Matching Criteria	Mean Age ± SD, Years (Range)	Mean Disease Duration for Control Group, Years (range)	Personality Measure(s) Used	Overall Findings
Not given	65.93 ± 4.17	Not given	TPQ	PD patients scored lower on novelty seeking and higher on harm avoidance than controls. PD patients treated for depression scored even higher on harm avoidance than PD patients who were not treated with antidepressants.
Age and sex	44.5 ± 4.6 (31–50)	Not given	German version of the TPQ	PD patients scored higher than controls on harm avoidance and reward dependence, specifically the subscale persistence.
Part I: Age Part II: NA	Part I: 59.8 ± 8.7 (40–74) Part II: NA	Part I: NA Part II: NA	Part I: TCI and the Karolinska Scales of Personality (KSP) Part II: 6-[^{18}F]fluoro-l-dopa PET with MRI coregistration	Part I: PD patients scored higher on the TCI scale harm avoidance and the KSP muscular-tension scale. Part II: Only a relationship between uptake in the right caudate and the TCI harm-avoidance scale was found.
Age and education	63.8 ± 10.1 (no range)	Not given	Hebrew version of the TPQ	PD patients scored lower on novelty seeking and higher on harm avoidance than controls. Right-onset PD patients scored lower on novelty seeking than controls, whereas left-onset PD patients scored no differently. Left-onset PD patients scored higher on harm avoidance than controls, but there was no difference among right-onset PD patients and controls. These findings are related to dopaminergic depletion.
Age	65.6 ± 7.4 (no range)	Not given	TCI	PD patients showed much higher levels of harm avoidance than controls and had greater ECF impairment (decrease in recall of early autobiographical memories).

Table 6.1
(continued)

Author and Date	Location	Population Studied	Mean Age ± SD, Years (Range)	Mean PD Duration, Years (Range)	Mean Hoehn–Yahr Stage (Range)	Medication Information	Control Group Studied
Twin Studies							
Duvoisin et al., 1981	USA	12 MZ twins; one of the pair a PD patient	64 (45–79)	9			
Ward et al., 1984	USA	20 MZ twins; one of each pair with PD		8			
Heberlein et al., 1998	Germany and Switzerland	15 German-speaking twin pairs discordant for PD; 6 MZ twin pairs (4 males); 9 DZ twin pairs (5 males)	MZ twins: 58 ± 17 (no range) DZ twins: 65 ± 33 (no range)	MZ twins: 8 ± 50 (no range) DZ twins: 6 ± 4 (no range)	Not given; only mean UPDRS score given; MZ twins = 33 (20–47); DZ twins = 19 ± 22 (5–37)	Not given	17 healthy controls (medical personnel and senior citizens; 10 males)

NA, not applicable; PD, Parkinson's disease; AD, Alzheimer's disease; PET, position emission tomography; MZ, monozyotic; DZ, dizygotic.
*The participants were twins, but there were no data on effects of twinship on personality, and so forth.

Menza et al., 1995; Tomer & Aharon-Peretz, 2004). Not surprisingly, these personality alterations of PD are associated with dopaminergic dysfunction. Menza and colleagues (1995) reported a significant correlation in a sample of midstage PD patients between social novelty seeking and [18F]fluorodopa uptake in the left caudate. Kaasinen et al. (2001), in contrast, reported that the novelty-seeking personality trait did not significantly correlate with [18F]fluorodopa uptake in any of the brain regions they studied. Instead, they found a highly significant positive correlation between right caudate [18F]fluorodopa uptake and the harm-avoidance trait in their sample of 47 PD patients. More recently, Tomer and Aharon-Peretz (2004) reported that patients with greater DA loss in the left hemisphere evidenced reduced novelty seeking, whereas patients with reduced DA in the right hemisphere reported higher harm avoidance than that of healthy controls.

Matching Criteria	Mean Age ± SD, Years (Range)	Mean Disease Duration for Control Group, Years (range)	Personality Measure(s) Used	Overall Findings
				PD patients were introverted
			Clinical interview about childhood and past personality of individual	The affected twin at age 8 was usually the leader and was more self-controlled; 10 years before onset the affected twin was less usually the leader, more nervous less adventurous.
Age and sex	63 ± 20 (no range)	Not given	Freiburg Personality Inventory (FPI-R) and a semistructured interview assessing premorbid lifestyle and personality (among other items)	Twins with PD scored lower than controls in "achievement orientation" and "extraversion," and they scored higher in "inhibitedness," "somatic complaints," and "emotionality."

In McNamara, Durso, and Harris (2007), we used an updated version of Cloninger's TPQ personality inventory called the Temperament and Character Inventory, or TCI, to study the agentic aspects of the self in PD. In addition to the three TPQ dimensions of personality mentioned earlier, the TCI also yields subscales of direct relevance to agency. These subscales include "persistence," "self-directedness," and "cooperativeness." Tse and Bond (2005) have shown (in healthy individuals) that a global measure of social adaptation is inversely correlated with the TCI harm-avoidance scale and positively associated with the cooperativeness scale scores. TCI subscale scores, in fact, predicted gaze and social interaction patterns in healthy volunteers. In a group of 35 unselected, midstage patients with PD, we (McNamara, Durso, & Harris, 2007) found that PD patients were significantly more likely to evidence harm avoidance compared with control subjects [PD mean = 15.1 (6.0), controls mean = 10.4 (5.4), $p = 0.01$]. PD patients were also marginally less likely to be self-directed [PD mean = 32.2 (5.5), controls mean = 36.0 (8.7), p = 0.07] or persistent [PD mean = 5.2 (1.9), controls mean = 4.2 (2.1), p = 0.07] compared with control subjects.

The PD Personality Traits Are Correlated with Executive Cognitive Deficits

In all of our studies of personality profiles of PD (e.g., McNamara, Durso, & Harris, 2007; McNamara, McLaren, & Durso, 2007; McNamara et al., 1992, 2003, 2006), we have found that some aspect of that profile was correlated with performance on executive function tests. Other groups have found the same correlation: personality traits of PD such as openness to experience and emotional stability are associated with executive function deficits such as performance on the Tower of London planning task (Volpato, Signorini, Meneghello, & Semenza, 2009).

How the Personality Traits Might Contribute to Psychiatric Syndromes of PD via Social Cognitive Processing Deficits

At the heart of many of the neuropsychiatric disorders of PD (e.g., apathy, depression, delusions, anxiety, etc.) lies an altered sense of self and of social cognition. The agentic self is central to social cognition and therefore is central to social interaction more generally. When internal cognitive and perceptual experiences are altered due to a weakly activated agentic self system and a hyperactive limbic system, social interactions are impaired as well. The combination of these cognitive/perceptual deficits and difficult social interactions contribute to psychiatric symptomatology as seen in some PD patients. This is not to say that psychiatric syndromes are caused by these social cognitive deficits, but rather, social cognitive problems intensify the difficulties the disease imposes on the patient and his family.

In fact, dysfunction in the agentic self system has repercussions for all kinds of internal cognitive and perceptual processing including processing of emotional memories. For example, as mentioned earlier, in a recent study of 34 patients with PD and 17 age-matched controls with chronic disease, we (McNamara, Durso, & Harris, 2007) found that PD patients evidenced higher harm avoidance, lower novelty-seeking scores, and lower recall rates of personally experienced events from childhood than that of controls, and this PD personality profile was associated with poorer performance on neuropsychological tests of prefrontal function. We also found that PD patients recalled fewer autobiographical memories in a 90-second interval than did controls. When we plotted the recall curve (see figure 6.1) as a function of 15-second intervals, we found that PD patients recalled a roughly similar

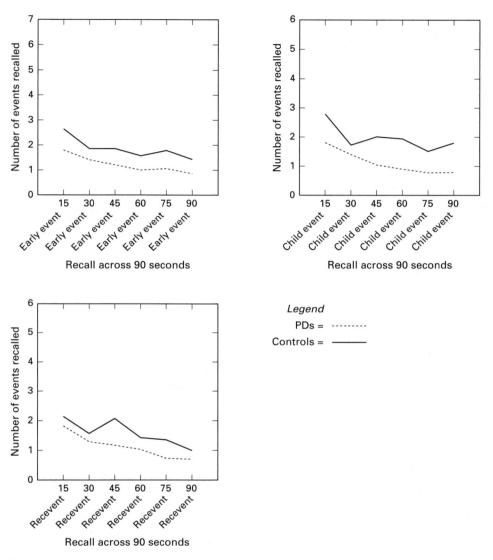

Figure 6.1
Autobiographical memory rates of recall per 15-second interval for early, childhood, and recent events in PD versus control groups. PDs, Parkinson's disease patients. (From McNamara, P., Durso, R., & Harris, E. 2008. Alterations of the sense of self and personality in Parkinson's disease. *International Journal of Geriatric Psychiatry*, 23(1), 79–84. Reprinted with permission.)

number of *recent* events in the first time interval as that of controls. PD patients did not seem to have inordinate difficulty initiating recall or rapidly retrieving *recent* events relative to controls. This was not the case when patients attempted to retrieve long-term autobiographical memories. Here, initiation was significantly slower relative to controls. PD patient performance, furthermore, declined steadily across the time intervals, whereas controls exhibited a similar gradual decline and then a sudden increase during the final time intervals—at least on the long-term memory tasks (early and childhood recall). These recall results indicate that PD patients have relatively normal access to the *current minimal self* and relatively poor access to autobiographical memory aspects of the self. To retrieve and to use autobiographical memories in service to current goals, one needs to control working memory resources for effortful search processes in long-term memories. However, the frontal dysfunction of PD degrades working memory capacity.

In the realm of social cognition, mental simulations are used to support so-called "mentalizing" functions (*theory of mind*, or ToM, interpersonal empathy, and perspective taking) that involve the ability to model the mental states of others. These mentalizing abilities are all functions of the agentic self in its interactions with others. Mentalizing abilities, that is, the ability to infer accurately what other people are thinking, intending, and desiring in common social situations, are impaired in PD and likely contribute significantly to neuropsychiatric syndromes of PD. If the mentalizing functions are indeed selectively vulnerable in PD, then PD patients will be at a severe disadvantage in interacting with others. The inability to identify rapidly and accurately intentions, meanings, desires, and beliefs of others forces the PD patient to either make guesses about the intentions/meanings of others or to take longer to think about and formulate replies to others or to simply withdraw from social interactions altogether.

Developing an adequate theoretical account of alterations in the agentic self in its social cognitive functions is of fundamental clinical and theoretical importance. Clinically, social cognitive/behavioral deficits in PD increase caregiver burden (Caap-Ahlgren & Dehlin, 2002; Edwards & Scheetz, 2002), reduce quality of life (Global Parkinson's Disease Survey Steering Committee, 2002), and may compromise complex decision-making capacities around long-term care. As we have seen, the personality profile of people at risk for PD (which influences social interactions, of course) furthermore may predate onset of overt extrapyramidal motor signs of PD by several years, and thus, selected social cognitive deficits may predict risk for disease severity.

Social Cognition

Social cognition involves processing of interpersonal and relational information and thus involves at a minimum interactions between self and other (Anderson & Chen, 2002; Baldwin, 2003; Decety, 2007; Decety & Grèzes, 2006; Josephs & Ribbert, 2003; Keysers & Gazzola, 2007; Lieberman, 2007; Uddin, Iacoboni, & Lange, 2007). One of the functions of the agentic self in its capacity to control plans, goals, and actions more generally is to mediate social interactions. To perform social actions, the agentic self must model the beliefs, intentions, desires, and thoughts of other minds or persons (Anderson & Chen, 2002; Baldwin, 2003; Decety, 2007; Decety & Grèzes, 2006; Josephs & Ribbert, 2003; Keysers & Gazzola, 2007; Lieberman, 2007; Uddin et al., 2007). A key aspect of social cognition is, therefore, the ability to infer other peoples' mental states, thoughts, and feelings. This is sometimes referred to as ToM or mentalizing ability. Given that mentalizing abilities both support and are supported by intact emotional and executive cognitive functions (Anderson & Chen, 2002; Baldwin, 2003; Decety, 2007; Decety & Grèzes, 2006; Josephs & Ribbert, 2003; Keysers & Gazzola, 2007; Lieberman, 2007; Uddin et al., 2007), and given further that emotional, personality, and executive functions are impaired in PD (Crucian et al., 2001; Kaasinen et al., 2001; Mathias, 2003; McNamara & Durso, 2003; McNamara, Durso, & Harris, 2007; McNamara, McLaren, & Durso, 2007; McNamara et al., 2003, 2006; Menza et al., 1993; Menza et al., 1995; Tomer & Ahazron-Peretz, 2004; Tse & Bond, 2005), I suggest that mentalizing abilities are impaired in PD as well relative to age-matched controls.

Social Functions in PD

Problematic social behaviors in PD patients have been documented repeatedly (Crucian et al., 2001; Mathias, 2003; Menza et al., 1993) and are a commonplace observation in the neurology clinic. In our clinical experience, for example, social deficits of PD involve social withdrawal, lack of interest and initiative in pursuing social interactions, inability to "read" emotional or facial expressions of others, personality and mood changes, sexual improprieties, ignoring doctor's orders/ suggestions, irresponsible use of money (e.g., gambling away the family's savings), and a strange insensitivity to the social, moral, and personal consequences of inappropriate social behaviors.

Theory of Mind/Mentalizing Performance in PD

It is unclear whether ToM abilities are significantly impaired in PD. Most studies of ToM abilities in PD involve relatively small numbers of participants and mostly report some amount of impairment on one or more ToM tasks (Bodden et al., 2010; Mengelberg & Siegert, 2003; Monnetta, Grindrod, & Pell, 2009; Péron et al., 2009; Saltzman, Strauss, Hunter, & Archibald, 2000; Yoshimura & Kawamura, 2005). Although most studies report ToM deficits in PD patients, the study populations were small in at least two of the studies; information is unavailable on another study. In the Mengelberg and Siegert (2003) study, 13 PD patients were impaired on 3 of 4 ToM tasks, and in the Saltzman et al. (2000) study, 11 patients with PD had difficulty with false-belief stories and the "spy" model ToM task. The Yoshimura and Kawamura (2005) study was published in Japanese. Its English abstract reported significant PD impairment on a ToM task. We have not yet been able to obtain an English summary of the detailed results of this study. Monetta et al. (2009) showed that some PD patients exhibit difficulty differentiating irony and a lie. Péron et al. (2009) failed to find any significant difference in ToM performance between early PD patients and healthy controls. There was also no difference in performance in the on-LD versus off-LD state. In a group of 27 later-stage PD patients, performance on the intention attribution question ("cognitive" ToM score) in the faux pas recognition task was impaired. Bodden et al. (2010) studied ToM abilities in a group of 21 PD patients. They found that PD patients scored lower on both an affective and cognitive ToM task. There is a clear need to assess ToM abilities in PD in an adequately statistically powered study.

Social Roles/Social Scripts

Mentalizing abilities are at a premium for nonroutine social interactions. For routine social interactions, in contrast, we can rely on our access to well-rehearsed social scripts to infer intentions and actions of others involved in these routine interactions. To study mentalizing abilities of PD patients systematically, it is therefore important to establish their abilities to access efficiently knowledge embedded in these overlearned, routine social scripts. We (Johnson & McNamara, 2007) asked 33 midstage PD patients and 14 age-matched controls to identify basic social actions, social roles, and social perspectives of actors in basic social scripts like ordering a meal at a restaurant, going to the doctor's office (D), going to a religious service (R), and so forth, as well as a control task [making a sandwich

(S)] that would not necessarily involve social interactions. We found that both patients and controls produced very few basic social actions for each script and a large number of subordinate actions. PD patients produced significantly fewer basic social actions for the ordering a meal script than that of controls. Participant roles (waiters, nurses, doctors, pastors/clergymen, etc.) were less often mentioned in the PD reports (6 total across scripts) than in control reports (10 total across scripts).

A Subgroup of Machiavellian Personality Types

The personality profile of PD, the mentalizing and social cognitive deficits, suggests that there might be personality subtypes in PD. We (McNamara, Durso, & Harris, 2007) asked a group of midstage PD patients to complete two personality inventories: the TCI (Cloninger, Svrakic, & Przybeck, 1993) and the MACH-IV (Christie & Geis, 1970) scales, the latter assessing the extent to which social interactions of the respondent are characterized by suspiciousness, defensiveness, and "Machiavellian" manipulatory interpersonal tactics. We found no significant differences in the mean total score on the MACH-IV between the PD group [65.0 (17.5)] and the elderly control group [62.0 (20.4)]. However, when we split the PD group into high Mach versus low Mach using the standard median split procedure performed in most studies with the MACH scales, we found that whereas the two PD groups did not differ significantly in terms of age, education, Hoehn–Yahr disease stage, mood functions, or Mini Mental State Exam (MMSE) scores, the high-Mach individuals scored significantly lower on the cooperativeness and self-directedness subscales of the TCI, thereby identifying a subgroup of patients whose social functioning is altered relative to controls and other PD patients.

High-Mach abilities should intersect at some point with high extraversion and high agentic personality traits. If there is a group of PD patients with high Mach scores, then it suggests that some patients retain at least one aspect of agentic personality functioning. We compared the abilities of this subgroup of (high-Mach) PD patients using the low-Mach group as a control group. We asked both groups to listen to a description of a fictitious individual we named "Tom" and then indicate whether they wanted to interact socially with this individual. Would they consider starting a business with him, loaning him money, being his roommate, having him as a confidante, having him as a partner on a debating team, and so forth. We used the original MACH-IV scale items to describe "Tom." "Tom believed that there was a sucker born every minute." "Tom believes that the best way to handle people is

Table 6.2
Willingness of high-Mach versus low-Mach individuals to associate with a high-Mach individual in various social situations

	High-Mach Patients (SD)	Low-Mach Patients (SD)	p Value
Partner in business	–0.88 (2.1)	–2.4 (1.1)	0.01**
Share apartment	–1.2 (2.2)	–1.9 (1.3)	0.24
Confidante	–1.2 (2.2)	–1.9 (1.4)	0.24
Member debate team	–1.4 (1.5)	–2.4 (.87)	0.022*
Employer	–0.82 (1.9)	–0.88 (1.8)	0.012*
Loan money	–0.11 (2.0)	–1.9 (1.6)	0.007**
Total advantages	5.5 (4.6)	2.9 (3.0)	0.057
Total disadvantages	7.6 (3.6)	8.0 (2.8)	0.69

Note: Willingness to interact with a high-Mach individual was indicated on a scale of –3 (very *unwilling*) to 0 (indifferent) to +3 (very *willing*). SD, standard deviation. *$p \leq 0.05$; **$p \leq 0.01$.
Source: From McNamara, P., Durso, R., & Harris, E. (2007). "Machiavellianism" and frontal dysfunction: Evidence from Parkinson's disease (PD). *Cognitive Neuropsychiatry*, *12*(4), 285–300. Reprinted with permission.

to tell them what they want to hear." "Tom believed that honesty was never the best policy"; and so forth. Tom, in short, was a high-Mach individual. We also asked patients to rate the overall advantages or disadvantages of interacting with Tom socially. Table 6.2 displays results of these analyses.

High-Mach individuals indicated that they were more willing to associate with "Tom," our fictitious high-Mach person, than were the low-Mach individuals. This was the case for all six social opportunities except sharing an apartment and having Tom as a confidante. High-Mach individuals also were marginally more inclined to believe that advantages accrued when associating with Tom [PD mean = 5.5 (4.6) vs. control mean 2.9 (3.0); p = 0.057]. It is important to note, however, that none of the high-Mach individuals indicated an enthusiasm in associating with Tom—all of their mean ratings fell below the 0 indifferent point. The high-Mach individuals were merely less averse to Tom than were the low-Mach individuals. These results, nevertheless indicate that there are some PD patients (the high-Mach individuals) who appear willing to interact with a person that is explicitly described as an untrustworthy individual.

Summary

The research to date on the personality profile of people at risk for PD and of PD patients themselves is one of relatively high anxiety, cautiousness, and harm avoidance even decades before onset of motor symptoms. The low novelty-seeking, high harm-avoidance profile persists into the clinical period itself. With the onset of motor symptoms, other cognitive deficits follow that complicate social interactions. Strategic access to autobiographical memory is impaired in PD. The sense of self undergoes a shift toward conformity and social avoidance as the disease progresses. The personality profile is also associated with some negative social mentalizing behaviors in some PD patients. These patients are more willing than controls to interact with an individual who was explicitly described to them as a manipulative, untrustworthy, and exploitative individual.

We suggest that the alterations in the sense of self, as well as the social behaviors of PD patients including the harm-avoidance profile and the apparent willingness of some patients to associate with a socially untrustworthy individual, may be related to failures in mentalizing abilities. If one finds it difficult to understand, imagine, or infer the intentions, desires, and thoughts of others, one may adopt a policy of avoidance and conformism. Failures in mentalizing may be related to a more fundamental deficit in generating mental simulations of states of mind of others and predicted effects of one's own actions and other's actions.

The fundamental problem is, I suggest, the weak activation in the agentic self system and the associated hyperactivity in the limbic–amygdalar circuits that are normally inhibited by the DLPFC, which mediates the agentic self system. This weak activation in executive systems may extend back to early life. This latter finding points to either genetic or epigenetic effects that render the individual vulnerable to the disease process that ultimately produces PD. Presumably, the individual starts out life with a low complement of DA. Rewarding effects of striatal–prefrontal DA are, therefore, less available to these individuals so they are less likely to smoke, do drugs, or to engage in risky behaviors, more generally. The weakly activated agentic self system promotes personality traits of cautiousness, reluctance to take the leader's role, low novelty seeking, and the like. This scenario, however, does not adequately explain the industriousness, high accomplishments, high intelligence, and achievement orientation of many PD individuals. My own feeling is that PD patients tend to be exceptionally intelligent individuals, and this intelligence explains their drive and accomplishments, but admittedly there are no controlled studies that can yet support this claim.

The weakly activated agentic self system, however, helps us to understand the personality profile associated with both premorbid PD and post-onset PD. It also helps us to understand social cognitive deficits of PD.

7 Evolutionary Perspectives on the Agentic Self, Its Neural Networks, and Parkinson's Disease

I have argued that PD represents a selective impairment in agentic aspects of the self system and that the agentic self system is mediated by specific neural circuits that run from dorsolateral and anterior prefrontal PFC down to the basal ganglia and back up again. The main function of the agentic self is to execute plans and voluntary actions. The personality characteristics most often associated with the agentic self are novelty seeking, openness to experience, self-directedness, a risk-taking bias, and extraversion. These, of course, are all the personality traits that are low, altered, or downregulated both in healthy persons and in those at risk for PD. When PD patients are put on DA agonists that act on limbic sites, these personality characteristics are temporarily reversed in favor of an impulsive self system. But, for the most part, the premorbid and post-onset personality profile of PD is one of low novelty seeking, high harm avoidance due to high anxiety levels, introversion rather than extraversion, and a bias for caution rather than risk taking. Notably, there are ecologic and evolutionary pressures that favor the appearance of these sorts of personality traits and their opposites, and we can learn something interesting about PD neuropsychiatry via investigation of its evolutionary associations.

Evolution of Personality Traits Linked to an Agentic Self

It should not be surprising that some ecologic contexts favor a risk-taking personality, whereas others favor a more cautious risk-averse personality. When risk taking is favored, there has to be physiologic mechanisms that can adjust dopaminergic activity levels upward to support risk-taking cognitions and behaviors. Conversely, when ecologic contexts demand a more risk-averse strategy, dopaminergic activity levels need to be adjusted downward to promote harm-avoidant strategies, reduced risk taking, and so forth. In people at risk for PD, the internal

DA-control thermostat appears to be set to promote a risk-averse orientation by increasing anxiety levels and harm-avoidant strategies at the expense of extraverted, novelty-seeking strategies.

That ecologic context can influence a range of personality traits is illustrated by several lines of evidence. Camperio Ciani, Capiluppi, Veronese, and Sartori (2007) showed that people whose families had inhabited a set of small islands for 20 generations or more scored lower on both extraversion and openness to experience than did the recent immigrants to the islands. The 7R allele of the DRD4 gene is known to be associated with novelty seeking and extraversion (Ebstein, 2006). Notably, it occurs at dramatically different rates according to ecologic context. It appears to increase in frequency when people migrate to new environments or inhabit resource-rich environments (Chen, Burton, Greenberger, & Dmitrieva, 1999; Penke, Denissen, & Miller, 2007). Migratory populations show a far higher proportion of long-allele DRD4 genes than do sedentary populations.

The long 7 repeats allele (L-DRD4) has also been identified in clinical and nonclinical populations with ECF deficits including set-shifting and sustained attention (Kieling, Roman, Doyle, Hutz, & Rohde, 2006), spatial working memory (Froehlicha et al., 2007), and verbal fluency deficits (Alfimova et al., 2007). These clinical populations very often score high on impulsivity scales. It is possible that the L-DRD4 enhances extraverted personality traits when individuals are young, but then these individuals find it harder to develop strategies to inhibit the impulsive traits they were born with, and thus, they perform poorly on ECF tasks as adults. Enhanced impulsivity in the context of ECF deficit can lead to severe behavioral disturbances in PD (Voon et al., 2007; Weintraub et al., 2006). Although persons at risk for PD and PD patients themselves are *not* characteristically impulsive, they can become so when they are put on DA agonists. Once this occurs, the individual has an activated limbic system in the context of severe ECF deficit, and thus, impulsive thinking and responding increases. Given the fact that persons at risk for PD are not impulsive and they are not typically sensation seekers or extraverted, one would predict that the L-DRD4 polymorphism would be rare in these individuals. If so, the absence of such an allele would constitute a biomarker for the premorbid personality type discussed above and in previous chapters. It would further imply that incidence of PD would vary in an inversely proportional way with the frequency of the L-DRD4 polymorphism. Where L-DRD4 occurred, one would predict reduced incidence of PD. But, not surprisingly, matters are a bit more complex than these simple predictions. Nevertheless, the relationships among L-DRD4, the "PD personality" type, and PD risk are worth exploring a bit more in depth.

DRD4 Variants and PD

The dopamine-four-receptor (DRD4) is a metabotropic, G protein–coupled receptor that has been classified as a D_2-like receptor. The D_2 class of receptors all function to inhibit adenylyl cyclase (Oldenhof et al., 1998). DRD4 contains four exons that encode a 387-amino-acid protein with 7 transmembrane domains, an N-linked glycosylation site, and numerous phosphorylation sites (Van Tol et al., 1991). DRD4 is differentially expressed across varied regions of the brain, with the PFC containing the highest density of these receptors (Dulawa, Grandy, Low, Paulus, & Geyer, 1999). Additionally, high expression of DRD4 markers has been detected in the medulla, midbrain, and amygdala (D'Souza et al., 2004). DRD4 demonstrates an unusually high number of polymorphisms across the human species. Variability includes single-nucleotide polymorphisms (SNPs) and variable numbers of tandem repeats (VNTR). The most studied polymorphism is a VNTR in exon III of DRD4. The most common variants are the 2-repeat VNTR (2R VNTR), 4-repeat VNTR (4R VNTR), and 7-repeat VNTR (7R VNTR) accounting for more than 90% of all DRD4 polymorphisms. Across demographic classes, the 4R VNTR is the most common variant. 2R polymorphs are a more common minor variant in Asian cultures, and the 7R allele is the most frequent minor variant in Western cultures (Chang, Kidd, Livak, Pakstis, & Kidd, 1996).

Ricketts et al. (1998) demonstrated an association between PD and long variants of the VNTR in exon III of DRD4. Juyal et al. (2006) found an association between DRD4 120-bp duplication markers and PD among the peoples of both the northern and the southern Indian subcontinent (Juyal et al., 2006). In the Ricketts et al. study, approximately 45% of the 95 PD patients they studied contained at least one allele longer than the 4R, such as the 7R, 8R, or 10R. This is a significant finding given that the frequency of the 7R allele is approximately 13% in North American healthy participants (Comings et al., 1999). Kronenberg et al. (1999), however, found no association between the allele and a group of German PD patients. Wan et al. (1999) also failed to detect a correlation between DRD4 polymorphisms of exon III and a group of 101 Chinese PD patients. There was only 3.4% frequency of 7R alleles in this population sample.

DRD4 polymorphisms have also been implicated in sleep attacks in PD. Paus et al. (2004) found that PD patients with 2R and 7R variants were more likely to suffer from sleep attacks compared with PD participants without these variants. However, Rissling et al. (2004) found no association between sleep attacks in PD and any variants of DRD4.

The available data on DRD4 polymorphisms in the PD population do not allow us to conclude our prediction that the incidence of PD should be in inverse proportion to the frequency of the long repeat variant of the gene. The logic of this prediction, however, is simple: the L-DRD4 polymorphism is a marker for extraverted and novelty-seeking personality types, but people at risk for PD typically exhibit a profile of personality traits that are exactly opposite that of the extraverted, novelty-seeking personality. That agentic component of the personality system is targeted by the disease process and so it is reduced or absent in people at risk for PD, and to that extent, the genes that make the risk-taking novelty-seeking personality type possible should be silenced or their activity attenuated in people at risk for PD.

The agentic self system that is the target of the disease process in PD is mediated by the DLPFC and anterior PFC in interaction with their subcortical targets in the basal ganglia. To what extent can we discern a specific evolutionary history for this sector of the massive human PFC?

Evolution of Prefrontal Networks Subserving the Agentic Self

The PFC constitutes approximately one third of the human cortex and is the last part of the human brain to become fully myelinated in ontogeny, with maturation occurring in late childhood/early adolescence (Huttenlocher & Dabholkar, 1997). In humans, the frontal lobes mediate what are believed to be distinctively human mental capacities such as language generativity (Corballis, 2002;), autobiographical memory retrieval (Wheeler, Stuss, & Tulving, 1997), ToM (Saxe & Baron-Cohen, 2006), empathy (Adolphs, Tranel, Damasio, & Damasio, 1994), working memory (Goldman-Rakic, 1987), executive functions (Delis, Kaplan, & Kramer, 2001), impulse control (Ray & Strafella, 2010), volition (Passingham, 1993), and possibly, as I have been arguing in this book, even the agentic sense of self (Vogeley et al., 2004).

How does the brain evolve new circuits or networks that can support such complicated functions as an agentic, or executive, self system—an emergent "system" that identifies values, chooses among them, makes decisions, inhibits impulses, formulates plans by constructing counterfactual mental simulations, and pursues goals, and so forth.? On the model of *mosaic evolution* (Barton & Harvey, 2000; Holloway, 1968), evolutionary forces can act on individual interconnected neural circuits that mediate specialized behavioral capacities without altering overall brain size. In this model, individual circuits can change in size in relative independence of changes in overall brain size. This model can be tested by looking for correlations between structures linked by important functional and anatomic connections that remain after accounting for the effects of size change in other structures (i.e., analysis of *correlated evolution* of individual functional sites). Alternatively, the *developmental constraints* model of brain evolution (Finlay & Darlington, 1995; Finlay, Darlington, & Nicastro, 2001) postulates that a single mechanism (e.g., genes regulating prenatal neocortical development) act to produce a generalized effect on the absolute size of all brain regions. Genetic changes, for example, could prolong the division of progenitor cells that give birth to neocortical neurons (Rakic, 1995), which would subsequently increase the size of the forebrain, generally. Finlay and Darlington (1995) factor-analyzed the covariances among the absolute size of 12 brain regions across 131 species of mammals and found that a single factor accounted for 96% of the variance, thereby supporting the single developmental mechanism theory of brain evolution. Finlay and Darlington's methods and conclusions, however, have been criticized by a number of authors (see commentaries in Finlay et al., 2001), and thus, the theory remains controversial.

PFC evolution must be seen against the background of neocortical evolution. Variation in neocortical size and structure is best exemplified among the primates. Anthropoid primates typically have larger neocortices for their body size (Stephan & Andy, 1969) or for their brain size (Radinsky, 1975) relative to prosimians. Human neocortex is 2.9 times larger than expected for an anthropoid primate of the same body size (Passingham, 1973). When neocortical volume is compared against total brain volume, however, humans' neocortical size does not depart significantly from expected values for non-human primates of similar brain size (Passingham & Ettlinger, 1974). Deacon (1990) has argued that some of these conclusions concerning neocortical size in humans are biased because one variable in the analysis (the neocortex) constitutes between 60% and 80% of the variance of the variable it is plotted against (brain weight or brain volume). The issue of relative neocortical size in humans compared with other primates remains unresolved. The regional pattern of gyrification across the brain has also been compared in several species (Zilles, Armstrong, Moser, Schleicher, & Stephan, 1989; Zilles, Armstrong, Schleicher, & Kretschmann, 1988). The largest discrepancy between pongid and human gyrification is in the PFC, where the human brain appears to be uniquely "gyrified."

Evolutionary History of the PFC in Mammals

The PFC is defined in modern neurobiology by its connections with other cortical sites and with subcortical sites. There are variations among species in the pattern of connections between PFC and subcortical and cortical sites, but within the mammalian class of animals, a broad generalization is tenable: The PFC is that expanse of cortex that is reciprocally interconnected with the dorsomedial nucleus of the thalamus. Defined in this manner, we observe that in most *primates,* three broad subdivisions have been identified: dorsal, mesial, and orbitofrontal divisions. In other mammals, such as the common laboratory rat, only two major subdivisions can unambiguously be identified: the orbitofrontal division and a mesial division deriving from the ACC (Preuss, 1995). No lateral division exists. Nevertheless, available evidence suggests that PFC can be identified in all extant mammals studied to date. Some portion of PFC (the orbito or mesial division) has even been identified in monotremes (Johnson, 1990) and in marsupials (Benjamin & Golden, 1985). Indeed, some authors have claimed that the PFC in at least one monotreme (the echidna) is disproportionately larger relative to body size than the PFC is in humans (Divac, Holst, Nelson, & McKenzie, 1987; Divac, Pettigrew, Holst, & McKenzie, 1987). In humans, the frontal lobes comprise the large expanse of cortex in the anterior portions of the brain (Banyas, 1999; Fuster, 1989; Goldman-Rakic, 1987). They are not fully myelinated until the adolescent or adult years. They receive projections from the mediodorsal nucleus and give rise to primary motor cortex, as well as premotor, supplementary motor, and prefrontal (proper) areas. All of these areas send inhibitory efferents onto their sites of termination. The motor–premotor areas comprise Brodmann areas 4, 6, parts of area 44 (Broca's area), and the frontal eye fields. The paralimbic cortex of the anterior cingulate region merges with orbitofrontal cortex—a region implicated in emotional, reward, and social regulation. A dorsolateral/anterior prefrontal region includes Brodmann areas 9, 10, 11, 12, 45, 46, and 47 and is implicated in planning, mental simulation, delayed responding, and language functions. This is the system theorized to undergird the agentic self. It becomes very clearly delineated only in humans, but its precursors are evident in primates as well, especially the great apes.

PFC in Primates

Size Differences

Much of the comparative work on the PFC has (understandably) focused on the question of the relative size of the PFC in humans compared with that in other primates. These studies, however, have produced conflicting results, with some claiming substantial disproportionate increases in human PFC (Blinkov & Glezer, 1968;

Rilling & Insel, 1999) and others reporting little, if any, relative increases (Uylings & van Eden, 1990). Methodological differences including controversy over how best to demarcate PFC boundaries on specimens or on brain scans may explain some of these discrepant findings. Given the well-known problem of postmortem brain shrinkage, investigators have turned to MRI as a more reliable method for analysis of volumetric differences in animals. Schenker, Desgouttes, and Semendeferi (2005) analyzed MRI brain scans of 10 human and 17 ape subjects and reported that the PFC dorsal sector was the largest of the three sectors of the frontal cortex, with individual volumes ranging from 29.6 to 66.5 cm^3 in great apes, 7.2 to 8.3 cm^3 in gibbons, and 137.7 to 191.5 cm^3 in humans. The second largest was the mesial sector, and the smallest subdivision was the orbital sector. Semendeferi et al. (1997) measured the three frontal sectors in a small sample of postmortem primate brains (one of each for the chimpanzee, gorilla, orangutan, and gibbon) and in four living humans. They reported that the orbital sector of the frontal lobe was relatively smaller in the orangutan compared with that in other great apes (but this was based on only a single subject). The PFC, considered with its underlying white matter, was not larger than expected for primates of similar brain size. Noting that previous studies that reported greater relative PFC volumes in humans compared with those in other species were based on small sample sizes with little representation from the great apes (our nearest relatives), Semendeferi et al. (2002) analyzed MRI brain scans of 24 non-human primates including 15 great apes, 4 gibbons, and 5 monkeys, as well as 10 healthy humans. They found no evidence for disproportionate enlargement of human PFC relative to the great apes. Schenker et al. (2005) found that the size of the dorsal sector as a percentage of the frontal lobe separated the two *Pan* species (chimps and bonobos) and was relatively larger in chimpanzees than in bonobos. In spite of having the largest brains among the great apes in their sample, orangutans had some of the smallest values for the orbital sector in terms of absolute size thus replicating an earlier finding (Semendeferi et al., 1997). But, again, Schenker et al. found no evidence of disproportionately large PFC in humans. Nevertheless, Semendeferi et al. have reported positive allometry for at least one area within the PFC: Brodmann area 10 (BA10). Recall that this is a region that I have argued, on the basis of behavioral data, to be crucial for the agentic self. Similarly, Bush and Allman (2004) analyzed a series of MRI scans of postmortem tissue/brain slices of various neural regions from 25 primate species and 15 carnivore species. They reported that humans have a PFC commensurate with that of an ape the size of an average human. Lemurs, gibbons, chimpanzees, and other primates have roughly the same proportion of brain tissue devoted to the frontal cortex as people do (roughly 36% of brain volume), but lions, hyenas, and other carnivores display evidence of a smaller frontal cortex (roughly 30%) relative to the rest of the brain. Intriguingly, in contrast to the above reports of Semendeferi et al., lemurs and other prosimians evidenced a slightly *greater* frontal cortex proportion than that of people and great apes. In summary, apart from the potential exception of BA10, size does not pick out what is distinctive about human PFC. Perhaps connectivity patterns are more important.

Connectivity Differences

Cortical white matter increases disproportionately with increasing brain size across mammals (Ringo, 1991), and therefore, it might also in primates. Zhang and Sejnowski (2000) derived a scaling law from an analysis of white and gray cortical matter in 59 mammals. They reported that a single power law of 4/3 captures the relationship between the volume of neocortical gray matter and the volume of adjacent white matter. Primates with larger brains tend to have an increased ratio of white to gray matter relative to other mammals indicating, perhaps, selection on brain circuits processing traffic between sites rather than on regional structures themselves. Schoenemann, Sheehan, & Glotzer (2005) analyzed gray matter, white matter, and total volumes for both prefrontal and total cortex on 46 high-resolution MRI scans of individuals from 11 primate species: 12 *Homo sapiens*, 4 *Pan paniscus*, 6 *Pan troglodytes*, 2 *Gorilla gorilla*, 4 *Pongo pygmaeus*, 2 *Hylobates lar*, 4 *Cerco-cebus torquatus atys*, 2 *Papio cynocephalus*, 3 *Macaca mulatta*, 3 *Cebus paella,* and 4 *Saimiri sciureus*. They found that prefrontal percentage white matter in *Homo sapiens* was significantly different from that in all species except *Gorilla gorilla* and *Cebus apella*, whereas prefrontal percentage gray matter differed significantly only from that in *Macaca mulatta, Cercocebus torquatus atys, Cebus paella,* and *Saimiri sciureus*. The lack of statistically significant differences between *Homo sapiens* and *Gorilla gorilla* may partly be due to the fact that only two *Gorilla* brains were available. When non-human primate individuals were pooled into the taxonomic categories of Hominoidea (apes: *Pan paniscus, Pan troglodytes, Gorilla gorilla, Pongo pygmaeus, Hylobates lar*), Cercopithecoidea (Old World Monkeys: *Cercocebus torquatus atys, Papio cynocephalus, Macaca mulatta*), and Platyrrhini (New World Monkeys: *Cebus apella, Saimiri sciureus*), *Homo sapiens* was signifi-cantly different from these groups in prefrontal percentage total cerebrum and prefrontal percentage white matter. Some evidence for positive allometry of PFC white matter was found: prefrontal white matter volume in humans was significantly larger than predicted.

Summary

These examples of variation in size and structure of the frontal lobes in animals from the monotremes to primates reveal a trend in the primates that is most marked in great apes and humans for increasing connectivity in the dorsal PFC sector—the sector that I have argued subserves the agentic self.

Evolutionary Cytoarchitectonic Theory

One way to conceptualize the evolution of this dorsal sector of the PFC is in terms of evolutionary cytoarchitectonic theory. Based on the study of comparative cortical architecture, Sanides (1964, 1970, 1972) and Pandya, Seltzer, and Barbas (1988) proposed that the cerebral cortex of higher mammals develops in evolution by progressive elaboration of two primordial structures: the amygdala and the hippocampus. It will be seen that in our terms, the trend associated with the amygdala supports emergence of the minimal self, whereas the trend associated with the hippocampus supports the emergence of the agentic self. Pandya and others (Pandya & Seltzer, 1982; Pandya et al., 1988; Petrides & Pandya, 1999, 2002) have subsequently demonstrated that the dual origin of the cerebral cortex, as proposed by Sanides, is preserved in the connectional anatomy of the cerebral cortex. Specifically, each of the two primordial moieties give rise to a series of interconnected nuclei that preserve relationships with preceding structures in the series and ultimately with the root (amygdala vs. hippocampus) structure.

Proceeding from the oldest and most primitive three-layered configuration in the primordial limbic zones—referred to as allocortex—one passes through transitional periallocortical and pro-isocortical stages (paralimbic areas), to the newest and most fully developed six-layered cortex known as isocortex (or neocortex). A ventral system, arising from the amygdala and adjacent olfactory cortex, includes ventral portions of the frontal, parietal, and occipital lobes, the insular lobe, and most of the temporal lobe. Functionally, it is specialized for identifying stimuli, elaborating emotional responses to stimuli, and supporting the motivational aspects of behavior. The dorsal system arises from the hippocampal cortex and includes the dorsolateral surfaces of the frontal, parietal, and occipital lobes, basal ganglia, portions of the cingulate gyrus, and the adjacent parahippocampal gyrus. It is specialized for representing the spatial environment and organizing action in time and space. Notably, as the dorsal-medial trend progresses, pyramidal cells are increasingly prominent, whereas the ventral-lateral trend emphasizes granular cells.

The dorsal and ventral systems are in mutual inhibitory balance in order to support optimal functioning of the organism. If the evolutionary cytoarchitectonic model of PFC evolution is correct, then the evolution of the neural network that supports the agentic self emerged out of the dorsal trends, and it is not surprising that the neural networks that support the agentic self are densely interconnected with the basal ganglia, hippocampal, and parahippocampal sites. Nor is it surprising that the agentic system acts to inhibit the structures of the ventral system including the amygdala.

Pribram and McGuiness (1975) presented a similar neural model of what I have been calling the agentic self that is consistent with the evolutionary data summarized above. They postulated two separate neural networks extending from the neurotransmitter nuclei in the brain stem and other subcortical sites up to PFC sites in each hemisphere. Right-sided networks act to decrease their firing with repetitive input while left-sided sites increase their firing in response to continued stimulation. An "arousal" system produces a phasic response to repetitive input while an "activation" system maintains tonic readiness for action. The arousal system is based on the amygdala and on right-hemisphere networks. It is a novelty-seeking system. Thus, repetitive stimulation produces habituation in this system. The system prefers norepinephrine and serotonin as its neuromodulators. In contrast, the activation system is regulated by connections to the basal ganglia and prefers DA and acetylcholine as its neuromodulatory transmitters. Notably, Pribram and McGuiness suggest that the sense of "effort" reflects hippocampal activity that regulates the balance between the arousal and activation systems.

What all these evolutionarily inspired models of the neural systems that support agentic control and action more generally tell us is that the dorsal PFC–basal ganglia loops that support the agentic self are relatively recent innovations in the evolutionary story and they both support prospective action and the inhibition of impulsive responding. The postulation of a set of neural systems that support something that resembles what I have been calling the agentic self is plausible given the evolutionary and comparative data summarized above. Unfortunately, the evolutionary anatomy does not tell us why the agentic system is targeted in PD. That crucial piece of information will need to wait for the results of future research. If, as we argued above, chaotic ecologic environments promote a facultative shift from a risk-seeking to a risk-averse behavioral strategy; and if, further, people with PD generally adopt risk-averse behavioral strategies or personality traits, then it may be that people with PD were at one time exposed to environments that promoted a facultative shift into a risk-averse biobehavioral strategy that would then exacerbate any physiologic vulnerability or insult associated with degeneration in dopaminergic cell groups. Conversely, placing these people in less chaotic environments or in some way assisting them in developing strategies that would act to reduce the extreme risk-aversion behavioral orientation they operate under might help to ameliorate some of the associated behavioral effects of PD.

I have been arguing that the core cognitive deficit of PD is a weak activation of the agentic self system that is mediated by striatal–DLPFC and frontopolar cortical networks. This failure to fully activate the agentic self leads to hyperactivity in the minimal self system, which is subserved by limbic and orbitofrontal networks. The imbalance of activation between the agentic and the minimal self systems ultimately contributes to the executive control cognitive deficits of PD and the disabling symptoms of the neuropsychiatric disorders of PD (as I will discuss in the chapters on neuropsychiatric syndromes of PD). Recent studies of language functions in PD are consistent with the idea of a weakly activated agentic self system in PD. I will argue that these language deficits of PD are best understood as an inability to use language efficiently to accomplish actions.

Characterization of the Language Deficit in PD

Patients with PD exhibit inordinate difficulties in what is called the *pragmatics* component of language. Pragmatics concerns the appropriate use of language to accomplish actions in appropriate contexts. In recent studies of pragmatic abilities of patients with PD, we (Holtgraves & McNamara, 2010a,b; Holtgraves, McNamara, Cappaert, & Durso, 2010; McNamara & Durso, 2003; McNamara, Holtgraves, Durso, & Harris, 2010) found that patients with PD were significantly impaired on everyday use of language to accomplish actions. To assess pragmatic competence, we presented the patient with a series of prescripted, open-ended questions in an attempt to elicit as much casual conversation as possible. We used the validated Prutting and Kirchner (1987) checklist of core pragmatic skills to score the patient's conversations to see whether patients used a variety of pragmatic indicators, including *speech acts*, in an appropriate manner. Speech acts are crucial here as they constitute a direct index of people's ability to use language to perform actions. The five major types of speech acts are (1) *representatives* (e.g., asserting, claiming, concluding, reporting, and stating); (2) *directives* (e.g., advise, command, order, question, and request; in using a directive, the speaker tries to get the listener to do something); (3) *commissives* (e.g., offers, pledges, promises, refusals, and threats; here the speaker commits himself to a future course of action); (4) *expressives* (e.g., apologizing, blaming, congratulating, praising, and thanking); and (5) *declarations* [e.g., pronouncing ("I now pronounce you man and wife"), bidding, declaring, excommunicating, firing/dismissal, and nominating].

When we tallied both appropriate and inappropriate instances of speech act productions/comprehension as well as all the other categories on the Prutting and Kirchner checklist of pragmatic indicators, we found that patients with PD were significantly impaired (scored as inappropriate) on 20.4% of the items (a mean of 6 items per patient), whereas controls were "inappropriate" on only 3.8% of items. Although simple speech acts were produced, they were often used inappropriately, and the number and variety of speech acts were reduced relative to control participants. In short, PD patients experience inordinate difficulty using those components of language that are specifically designed to accomplish actions. More specifically, they experience inordinate difficulties producing and comprehending speech acts. I will review experimental evidence for this assertion later, but first I will briefly explain what speech acts are and why they are important for both linguistic theory and for PD.

Speech Acts and Pragmatics

Speech act theory (Austin, 1962; Searle, 1969) has been a very influential approach to language use and has a richly developed research base in the areas of analytic philosophy and logic (Grice, 1989; Searle & Vanderveken, 1985), artificial intelligence (Cohen & Levesque, 1990), psychology (Clark, 1996; Gibbs, 1999), and computational linguistics (Cohen, Morgan, & Pollack, 1990). As noted by Bara, Tirassa, and Zettin (1997), speech acts are a particularly useful tool for neuropsychological investigations of language use as they function to carry speaker intentions.

Implicatures are intentions or meanings implied by a speaker who utters a phrase designed to get the listener to do something. Patients with PD also evidence deficits in processing implicatures (see later) possibly because it would require them to comprehend and perform the action involved. Grice (1975) distinguished between generalized and particularized implicatures. The former are implicatures that arise without the need for any reference to the context. That is, their meaning tends to be recognized regardless of the context of the remark. For example, metaphors (e.g., "My job is a jail"), idioms (e.g., "He spilled the beans"), and conventional indirect requests (e.g., "Can you open the window?") can usually be interpreted independent of any discourse context (Gildea & Glucksberg, 1983; Glucksberg, Gildea, & Bookin, 1982; Keysar, 1989). Particularized implicatures, in contrast, are completely context dependent and cannot be generated without reference to the context within which the utterance occurs.

One of the most basic dimensions of speaker meaning—illocutionary force—can be viewed as a generalized implicature. Illocutionary force, as defined by speech act theorists (e.g., Searle, 1969), is the action (e.g., thank, apologize, promise, etc.) a speaker intends to have recognized with an utterance. For example, when Bob says to Andy "I'll definitely do it tomorrow," he would generally be regarded as having performed the act of promising. Note that illocutionary force is often conveyed without use of the relevant speech act verb (e.g., the verb *promise* is not part of "I will definitely do it tomorrow"). It is in this way that illocutionary force often represents a (generalized) implicature.

Examples of illocutionary acts include accusing, apologizing, blaming, congratulating, giving permission, joking, nagging, naming, promising, ordering, refusing, swearing, and thanking. The functions or actions just mentioned are also commonly referred to as the illocutionary force or point of the utterance.

As mentioned above, when we observed and quantitatively tallied pragmatic communication skills in conversations of PD patients, we noticed a significant difficulty with speech act production and comprehension. We therefore decided to investigate speech acts processing more closely in a series of experiments summarized below.

Experimental Findings on Speech Act Production and Comprehension in PD Patients

The purpose of the initial set of experiments was to examine the comprehension of speech acts. If the agentic self relies on speech act processing to accomplish actions in everyday contexts, then patients with PD need to process efficiently the speech act utterances of others. One needs to be able to do this to act appropriately in social contexts and to formulate one's own actions in response to others. In experiment 1 (see Holtgraves & McNamara, 2010a,b; Holtgraves, McNamara, Cappaert, & Durso, 2010), participants (both PD patients and control participants) read short scenarios or stories of conversational interactions (see tables 8.1–8.3) that ended

Table 8.1
Sample scenario and speech act manipulation

Cheryl and Dan have been married for 20 years.
Dan tends to be somewhat forgetful.
Today, Cheryl is sure Dan *didn't remember* (had forgotten) his dentist appointment.
They are eating *breakfast* (dinner) together when Cheryl says to Dan:
Cheryl: *Don't forget* (I'll bet you forgot) to go to your dentist appointment today.
Probe: Remind.

Note: The speech act version contained the italicized material; the control version was created by replacing the italicized material with the material in parentheses.
Source: From Holtgraves, T., & McNamara, P. (2010). Pragmatic comprehension deficit in Parkinson's disease. *Journal of Clinical and Experimental Neuropsychology*, *32*(4), 388–397. Reprinted with permission.

Table 8.2
Target utterances used in experiment 1

Speech Act	Utterance
Assertives	
Agree	You're right. It's wrong to experiment on animals.
Blame	It's all Mary's fault.
Remind	Don't forget to go to your dentist appointment today.
Guess	I don't really know, but would estimate around $100.
Deny	I did not take your chainsaw.
Correct	The proper way is to ask by saying "Why aren't we going to the park today?"
Introduce	Brad, this is my friend Charles.
Excuse	I have not been feeling well.
Expressives	
Thank	I appreciate your help so much. I couldn't have done it without you.
Apologize	I'm so sorry that I ruined your shirt.
Complain	I can't believe they raised their rates again. Cable just keeps on getting more and more expensive.
Brag	Fantastic. I caught a bigger fish than anyone else. I was super happy.
Congratulate	That's awesome. I'm so happy for you.
Compliment	I like your coat.
Directives	
Warn	Watch out, there's a lot of cops around. I almost got caught speeding.
Encourage	Don't stop now. You can do it.
Beg	Please, please, please let me play. I will do anything you want me to do.
Demand	The bank must pay for the fee.
Ask	What time is it?
Invite	Would you like to come over for dinner tomorrow night?
Commissives	
Threaten	If you don't stop I'll tell your parents and you'll be grounded.
Promise	I swear I will be neater after the weekend.
Offer	If you need some help, just give me a call.
Reassure	I want to make sure you know that we're definitely not moving. We're staying right here.

Source: From Holtgraves, T., & McNamara, P. (2010a). Pragmatic comprehension deficit in Parkinson's disease. *Journal of Clinical and Experimental Neuropsychology*, *32*(4), 388–397. Reprinted with permission.

Table 8.3
Target utterances used in experiment 2

Speech Act	Utterance
Assertives	
Agree	You're right. We do need to discount some of our items.
Blame	It's all Mary's fault.
Remind	Don't forget to stop at the store on your way home from work.
Deny	I did not delete any files.
Expressives	
Thank	I appreciate your help so much. We couldn't have done it without you.
Complain	I can't believe they're asking us to work more overtime. They just keep piling and piling it on.
Brag	I played in a tournament last week and did great—placed 2nd out of 180. I was super happy.
Compliment	Hi. I really like your new car. It's very nice.
Directives	
Warn	Watch out. There's a lot of ice on the roads. I almost slid off the road a couple of times.
Encourage	Don't stop now. You can do it.
Demand	You must take this steak back and bring me another.
Invite	Hi. Would you like to come to our picnic this weekend?
Commissives	
Threaten	If you don't stop your dog from coming over here, I'm going to call animal control and they'll take him away.
Promise	I swear I will be on time from now on.
Offer	If you need some help with it, just let me know.
Reassure	I want to make sure you know that I'm definitely not planning on leaving. I plan on staying with this company.

Source: From Holtgraves, T., & McNamara, P. (2010a). Pragmatic comprehension deficit in Parkinson's disease. *Journal of Clinical and Experimental Neuropsychology*, *32*(4), 388–397. Reprinted with permission.

with an utterance that either performed a specific speech act (brag, beg, promise, etc.) or was a carefully matched utterance that did not perform that specific speech act (control). After indicating comprehension of the utterance, participants performed a timed lexical decision task. On critical trials, the target was a word naming the speech act performed with the prior utterance.

Results showed that lexical decision accuracy was high for both control and PD (see table 8.4 below) participants, indicating that PD participants were quite capable of performing this task when the target utterances were not speech acts. If, however, comprehension required speech act activation, PD performance declined. To perform the tasks accurately, lexical decisions had to be faster for the targets after the speech act utterances than after the control utterances. The critical finding was a significant Group X Speech Act Activation interaction. Consistent with past research, nonimpaired participants performed this task significantly more quickly when the target string was the speech act associated with the preceding utterance. In contrast, patients with PD did not demonstrate this effect (see table 8.4), suggesting that speech act activation is slowed or is not an automatic component of comprehension for people with PD. In addition, the size of this deficit was related to disease severity.

The experiment 1 results do not mean necessarily that PD patients cannot recognize the speech acts, only that it does not occur as efficiently or as rapidly as for control participants. The purpose of experiment 2 was to examine whether PD participants display a speech act recognition deficit if given unlimited time to make their decision. Hence, in experiment 2, participants were given unlimited time to indicate their recognition of the speech act performed with an utterance. Participants in this study read materials similar to those used in experiment 1. However, rather than performing a lexical decision task after utterance comprehension,

Table 8.4
Lexical decision accuracy by participant classification and speech act: Experiment 1

Group	Target Accuracy (%)		Target Verification Speed (ms)	
	Speech Act	Control Speech Act	Speech Act	Control Speech Act
PD	94.2	93.6	1,963	1,849
Control	93.4	96.0	1,266	1,368

Source: Modified from Holtgraves, T., & McNamara, P. (2010a). Pragmatic comprehension deficit in Parkinson's disease. *Journal of Clinical and Experimental Neuropsychology*, *32*(4), 388–397. Reprinted with permission.

participants instead were asked to provide a single word that they believed best described the action the speaker was performing with the prior remark. Participants were not under any time constraints; hence, this represents an off-line analogue of the experiment 1 task. PD participants identified significantly fewer speech acts (33.7%) than that of the control participants (47.9%). Even when given unlimited time to identify the speech act, PD participants identified only a third of the instances where the speaker performed an action with his speech, whereas controls identified half of such instances. Even when controls failed to identify the exact speech act in question, they named an act that was close to correct. This was not the case with the PD participants. The results of this experiment, therefore, demonstrate a deficit in speech act recognition in PD that is independent of temporal constraints. As in experiment 1, the size of this deficit was related to disease severity and executive cognitive deficits: The greater the severity of the motor and cognitive deficit, the greater the speech act recognition deficit, thus underlining the link between speech act processing and the agentic self system.

The purpose of these follow-up experiments was to examine the comprehension of particularized implicatures. To understand the actions of others and to formulate actions in response to those others, one needs to be able to compute particularized implicatures. That is, one needs to be able to identify intentions/actions of people even when they state them indirectly. In experiment 3, participants read question–reply exchanges. On the critical trials, the reply either did (indirect reply) or did not (control reply) violate the relevance maxim of Grice ("make your utterance relevant to the context"). When the reply violates the relevance maxim, it functions as an indirect reply conveying negative information. Often, people use indirect speech to avoid insulting others. If someone says "Did you like my speech?" and you answer "Public speeches are difficult to do well," you do not answer the question because you wish to avoid saying that you did not like the speech.

Returning to the experimental conditions, the control reply was identical to the indirect reply, but the preceding question was altered so that the reply was relevant for the question. After indicating comprehension of the reply, participants performed a sentence verification task. On the critical trials, the target was a paraphrase of the indirect meaning of the reply. If this indirect meaning is activated online, then participants should be faster at making this judgment when the target follows an indirect reply than when it follows a control reply. Sentence verification accuracy was high for both PD and control participants, and there was no difference between groups (see table 8.5). The critical finding was a significant Group X Target Type interaction. As can be seen in table 8.5, for control participants,

Table 8.5
Comprehending particularized implicatures: Experiment 3

Group	Target Accuracy (%)		Target Verification Speed (ms)	
	Indirect Reply	Control	Indirect Reply	Control
PD	92.0	97.0	2,356	2,306
Control	93.8	93.0	1,944	2,247

Source: From Holtgraves, T., & McNamara, P. (2010a). Pragmatic comprehension deficit in Parkinson's disease. *Journal of Clinical and Experimental Neuropsychology*, *32*(4), 388–397. Reprinted with permission.

sentence verification was enhanced when the target was an indirect interpretation of the preceding reply (303 milliseconds faster). PD participants, in contrast, did not show this effect (50 milliseconds slower). In this experiment, then, nonimpaired participants demonstrated online activation of the indirect meaning of indirect replies; the speed with which they verified targets was enhanced when the target was an indirect interpretation of the preceding reply. PD participants, in contrast, did not show this effect.

These results demonstrate a PD deficit for the online generation of particularized implicatures. It is possible, however, that PD participants could generate particularized implicatures if given enough time. This issue was explored in experiment 4. In this experiment, participants read scenarios describing situations (similar to those used in experiment 3) and question–reply exchanges in which the reply was either a disclosure or an opinion. The context was manipulated so that the requested information was described as clearly negative, clearly positive, or there was no information provided. Participants were asked to write down how they would interpret the reply, and those interpretations were coded in terms of valence (whether they indicated that the reply should be interpreted as conveying an opinion or disclosure, and if so, whether the conveyed information was negative, positive, or neutral). Participants overwhelmingly interpreted these types of replies as conveying negative information, and there was no difference between the no-context and the negative-context condition. Despite the fact that PD and control participants did not differ in the content of their interpretations, PD participants were significantly more confident in both their correct and their erroneous interpretations than were the control participants, thus demonstrating PD comprehension difficulty with grasping illocutionary force—even under nontimed, relaxed conditions.

The above experiments demonstrated significant speech act *comprehension* deficits in PD patients. We next investigated abilities of PD patients to *produce* an appropriate number and variety of speech acts.

The purpose of experiment 5 was to examine speech act production; that is, the ability of people to construct utterances that perform specific (implicit) speech acts. The general procedure was the reverse of experiment 2 (with different content). Participants read scenarios describing common situations and were asked to write down exactly what they would say to perform a particular speech act without using the word naming the act they were to perform. The utterances produced by participants were shown to a separate group of healthy participants (judgment group) who were asked to read each utterance and provide a one-word description of what each utterance is doing. The percentage of trials for which the intended speech act was identified served as the measure of speech act production. The speech acts produced by PD participants (24.1%) were recognized just as often as the speech acts produced by control participants (23.3%). Hence, PD participants did not demonstrate a deficit in the production of utterances designed to perform a specific speech act.

Successful language use, however, involves more than just the production of simple speech acts. This is because interpersonal considerations are salient, and speakers must fine-tune the form of their utterances based on these considerations. The interpersonal dimension of language has been captured well with the concept of politeness (Brown & Levinson, 1987). We next examined the ability of PD participants to vary the politeness of their remarks as a function of the context. Participants read scenarios in which they were asked to imagine being in certain situations in which they were to make a request or to give an opinion. Two variables were manipulated: degree of face-threat and relative status (i.e., boss, son, co-worker, etc.). The utterances generated by participants were coded (by two trained coders) in terms of politeness. For requests, PD participants produced utterances significantly less polite than those produced by control participants. More importantly, the politeness of requests varied as a function of face-threat (request size) for control participants but not for PD participants. For opinions, politeness varied as a function of status for control participants but not for PD participants. Hence, PD participants displayed a deficiency in modulating their politeness as a function of the context. Thus, whereas PD patients can produce simple speech acts in response to simple social scenarios, they are less able to produce complex speech acts (politeness) appropriate to more complex social contexts.

Our findings indicate that (1) online speech act activation is abnormal in PD; (2) online comprehension of particularized implicatures is abnormal in PD; and

(3) processing of indirect speech acts while observing politeness conventions is impaired in PD. All of these results suggest that PD patients may be at a disadvantage in using language to accomplish social action, particularly complex social actions. PD patients, however, do seem able to produce simple speech acts.

Other Speech and Language Deficits of PD Are Related to the Primary Deficit in Speech Act Processing

Speech Production

With regard to speech and language production, PD patients often exhibit fluency and motor speech disorders, word-finding difficulties, and hesitations and pauses at crucial points in an utterance (for review, see McNamara & Durso, 2000). Patients with PD may also sometimes exhibit varying degrees of dysarthria involving a reduction of speech volume and pitch. In terms of sentence production, even early-stage patients tend to use simplified sentence structures with an increase in the ratio of open-class items (nouns, adjectives) to closed-class items (determiners, auxiliaries, prepositions, etc.), as well as an increase in the frequency and duration of hesitations and pauses at critical sites in a sentence. Many PD patients exhibit inordinate difficulty in generating words to a target stimulus such as a letter or a semantic category (such as animals), and this fluency deficit is correlated with speech production deficits (McNamara et al., 1992). Longitudinal studies of cognitive change in PD have repeatedly shown that poor performance on semantic fluency tasks can be characteristic of the preclinical phase of cognitive disorders of PD and sometimes even dementia in PD (Bayles et al., 1996; Caparros-Lefebvre et al., 1995; Henry & Crawford, 2004; Jacobs et al., 1995; Levy et al., 2002; Stern et al., 1998; Troster & Woods, 2003; Waite, Broe, Grayson, & Creaset, 2001; Woods & Troster, 2003).

Processing of Verbs

PD patients exhibit greater difficulty in generating verbs versus nouns and in naming of actions than in naming of objects (Cotelli et al., 2007; Henry & Crawford, 2004). This discrepancy between action and object naming (Boulenger et al., 2008) may be due to dysfunction within the agentic self system (i.e., the DLPFC and frontopolar regions of the brain). These regions of the brain appear to mediate representation of action plans more generally (Gallese, Rochat, Cossu, & Sinigaglia, 2009; Shapiro et al., 2005), and thus impairment in these regions may influence processing of verbs as well.

In an extensive analysis of a corpus of PD conversations [using the Linguistic Inquiry and Word Count (LIWC) program; Pennebaker, Booth, & Francis, 2007], we (Holtgraves et al., 2010) documented a significant reduction in use of verbs and pronouns for patients with greater left-sided disease. Greater left-side severity was associated with use of fewer verbs and pronouns. In my view, this result is consistent with the idea that the agentic self system differentially depends on right PFC. Complementary analyses with right-side severity did not yield any significant effects, nor did using initial side of onset with symptoms as a predictor variable. Finally, additional exploratory analyses of the relationship between left-side severity and other LIWC categories yielded no significant differences; it appears the effects of left-side severity are relatively specific to verbs and pronouns.

Grammatical and Sentence Processing

With regard to language comprehension, PD patients often exhibit a mild to moderate sentence comprehension deficit (Angwin, Chenery, Copland, Murdoch, & Silburn, 2006; Arnott, Chenery, Murdoch, & Silburn, 2005; Colman, Koerts, van Beilen, Leenders, & Bastiaanse, 2006; Hochstadt, Nakano, Lieberman, & Friedman, 2006; Geyer & Grossman, 1994; Grossman, Carvell, Stern, Gollomp, & Hurtig, 1992; Grossman, Crino, Reivich, Stern, & Hurtig, 1992; Grossman, Stern, Gollomp, Vernon, & Hurtig, 1994; Grossman et al. 1991, 2001; Kemmerer, 1999; Lieberman, Friedman, & Feldman, 1990; Lieberman et al., 1992; McNamara, Clark, Krueger, & Durso, 1996; Natsopoulos et al., 1991, 1993; Terzi, Papapetropoulos, & Kouvelas, 2005; Whiting, Copland, & Angwin, 2005). Most of the authors of these studies suggest that impaired morphosyntactic performance in PD may, in part, be attributed to cognitive resource limitations (i.e., working memory and information processing speed). Automatic morphosyntactic processing routines remain relatively intact in PD (Friederici, Kotz, Werheid, Hein, & von Cramon, 2003; Longworth, Keenan, Barker, Marslen-Wilson, & Tyler, 2005), though, as we have seen, the exception is speech act recognition. Consistent with a link between grammatical deficits and the agentic self system, most of the grammatical processing deficits have been correlated with deficits in the domains of executive functioning (e.g., inhibition, cognitive flexibility, or set-switching) and working memory. The language deficits of PD, therefore, appear to be secondary to dysfunction in the agentic self system.

Data obtained from functional imaging studies are consistent with the general picture of a relatively intact automatic minimal self language system and an impaired effortful processing agentic self language system. Grossman et al. (2003), for example, demonstrated that patients with PD recruit different brain regions when performing sentence comprehension tasks than do controls. Compared with healthy participants, individuals with PD showed less striatal activation and reduced anteromedial prefrontal and posterolateral temporal activation when processing sentences with multiple embedded clauses. In addition, patients demonstrated increased activation of left temporoparietal and right frontal and posterior regions when processing these sentences. The enhanced activation in these brain regions is presumably due to the inability to achieve adequate activation in left prefrontal regions during sentence processing.

In summary, patients with PD demonstrate consistent deficits in speech act comprehension, verb production, and sentence processing—especially when the latter depends on executive control processes like working memory. These language processing deficits appear to be linked with dysfunction in DLPFC and executive dysfunction. In my terms, the language deficits are consistent with weak activation of the agentic self system.

Which comes first? Do the deficits in the language system lead to a weak agentic self or vice versa? How are these language processes bound up with the agentic self system and what are the consequences of these self and language deficits for neuropsychiatric syndromes of PD? To provide preliminary answers to these difficult questions, I will first discuss how agency structures language in general, and then I will discuss consequences of language dysfunction for the experience of self and mood.

Agency and Language Structure

Linguists, anthropologists, psychologists, and cognitive scientists have very frequently noted that all the world's languages are structured around the idea of the agent or agency. The structure of language has, at its core, a deictic origin of the I, here, and now (Ahearn, 2001; Comrie, 1981; Dixon, 1994), and all languages display grammatical devices to handle three basic relations involving the agent: *Subject* of an intransitive verb; *Agent*, or subject, of a transitive verb; and *Object* of a transitive verb.

Language most often involves actions, or in terms of social relations it is about "who did what to whom." These categories, "who," "did," "what," "to," and "whom," and so forth, are sometimes called thematic roles. The agent, or self, can take on a very specific range of theta roles. Its preferred role is *Agent*: this is the person who causes things to happen. But, the self also undergoes things as well. In this case, the self is on the receiving end of the action. This is the *patient* or *experiencer* role. The self can also be the owner of a thing or action (*possessor*) and the beneficiary of an action (*beneficiary*).

Languages the world over treat the self in rule-governed ways. In the majority of languages, the subjects of transitive (Agent) and intransitive verbs (patient, experiencer) are treated the same way syntactically, whereas the object of a transitive verb is treated differently. These languages are known as languages of the *accusative* type. When the opposite pattern obtains (e.g., the subject of a transitive verb is treated differently than the object of a transitive verb and the subject of an intransitive verb), the language is known as ergative. In these languages, agents are explicitly marked by some morphosyntactic device. In short, in accusative languages, Objects (placed in the accusative case) are treated differently from Subjects and Agents, whereas in ergative languages, Agents are treated differently from Subjects and Objects. In both language types, agents and agency are treated specially but with differing means.

The special status accorded to agency has pervasive effects on the grammar of languages and on cognitive and conceptual category processing as well. The special status accorded to agency places constraints on the concepts or nouns that can appear in the Agent position. Silverstein (1976) proposed an animacy hierarchy (figure 8.1) that moves from inanimate objects (common count nouns) to proper nouns to personal pronouns. The latter extend from third-person pronouns to

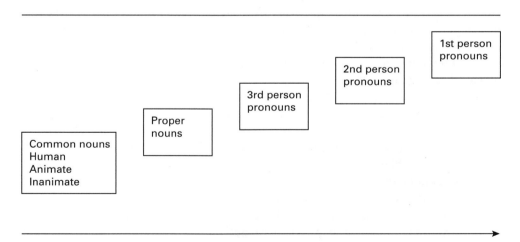

Figure 8.1
The animacy hierarchy from Ahearn, 2001. Reprinted with permission.

first-person pronouns. As one (or a language) moves from common nouns to first-person pronouns, eligibility for agency increases. The hierarchy also predicts where on the spectrum of noun phrases the split between ergativity and accusativity will occur. The items toward the right of the spectrum are more likely to be in the Agent function, and the items to the left of the spectrum are more likely to be in the Object position.

The structure of language therefore testifies to the centrality of the agent and action for human self-consciousness. Language itself likely evolved as a tool for the agent rather than as a medium that creates an agent. When we reflect on ourselves, we usually speak to ourselves. Our very thoughts are very often verbal or subvocal speech. When one uses the first-person singular personal pronoun *I*, it typically involves reference to one's bodily self at a specific point in time and space. That is, *I* is a deitic term—it is context dependent. The *I*, as a member of the class of personal pronouns, can also function anaphorically. It can refer back to or find its reference in a lexical entry from a previous utterance that names oneself. Because the first-person personal pronoun *I* can, according to the animacy hierarchy, embody the greatest amount of agency available in a language, changes in its use can be used to identify disorders of the self. For example, in children at risk for developing autism spectrum disorders, the appropriate use of *I* to refer to self rather than other either takes much longer than usual or is never consistently mastered. Similarly, in schizophrenia, *I* is not used normally by the patient during periods of active psychosis. In the narratives of people who are vulnerable to suicidal ideation, the use of *I* is paired with all kinds of negative content, and as we have seen earlier, the frequency of all personal pronouns declines in some PD patients.

To summarize major findings from this chapter: Patients with PD evidence significant language deficits, particularly in the realm of pragmatics, and within pragmatics, they have significant difficulty comprehending speech acts of all kinds and producing complex speech acts. Their problems with sentence processing appear linked with deficits in executive control processes like attention and short-term memory. I think it is reasonable to see the language deficits of PD as associated with their general problems in activating the agentic aspects of the self: the agentic self system (including the DLPFC, the ACC, and the rostral frontopolar PFC). Thus, the language deficits of PD can be considered in tandem with the array of cognitive deficits exhibited by patients with PD (reviewed in the previous chapters) as all pointing to the fundamental problem of adequately activating the agentic self system. I next examine the consequences of this disorder of the agentic self for manifestations of neuropsychiatric syndromes of PD.

In the past few chapters, we have been looking at the earliest predictors of PD. We have seen that an anxious personality in young adulthood significantly predicts risk for developing PD decades later. In middle age, a certain personality profile of anxiousness, harm avoidance, ambitiousness, inflexibility, punctuality, and reduced novelty seeking is also a significant predictor for later development of parkinsonism. Data uncovered in the past couple of decades have now shown that specific types of sleep disorders often develop 10–20 years before onset of motor symptoms of PD. That is, certain types of sleep dysfunction predict PD onset in some individuals about two decades later (see table 9.1).

From the point of view of the self, agentic and executive control systems come progressively under attack by the disease process that culminates in PD. There is an initial genetic, or epigenetic, vulnerability that weakens the agentic self system and manifests in generalized anxiety very early in life. This anxious trait then develops into a more consistent personality type in those individuals at risk for later development of PD. The premorbid personality type that sometimes precedes PD can be construed as a holding or defensive posture that accrues in the wake of a weakened agentic self system. If executive control processes are harder to mount and anxiety is more difficult to suppress, a consistent orientation toward risk or harm avoidance and reduced novelty seeking is not surprising. But why might a weakened agentic self system lead to sleep disorders?

The agentic self system is mediated by the prefrontal–subcortical loop as I have described in previous chapters. The DLPFC–basal ganglia–neostriatal loop inhibits and regulates the orbitofrontal–limbic–amygdalar loop that mediates the minimal self. We will see that it is the orbitofrontal–limbic–amygdalar loop that is activated each night during each rapid eye movement (REM) sleep period. Conversely, the DLPFC–subcortical loop is deactivated during REM sleep. In short, the agentic

Table 9.1
Risk factors in progression to PD

Risk Factor	Age
Elevated anxiety	Young adulthood
Premorbid personality profile (anxiousness, harm avoidance, ambitiousness, inflexibility, punctuality, reduced novelty seeking)	Middle age
Sleep disorders including RBD	10–20 years before onset of motor symptoms
Nonmotor and autonomic symptoms (constipation, loss of libido, loss of sense of smell, depression, various pain syndromes)	Decade before PD onset

self is silenced during REM sleep whereas the minimal self is activated. When this profile of activation/deactivation states is intensified due to disease-related impairment of the agentic self system, then the activation in the minimal self system becomes all the more intense and we get REM sleep behavior disorder (RBD). I will discuss RBD more thoroughly later. I begin by reviewing sleep disorders associated with PD and how they might contribute to neuropsychiatric symptoms associated with PD.

Sleep Dysfunction as a Source of Neuropsychiatric Disorder in PD

Sleep dysfunction contributes to a wide range of neuropsychiatric symptoms and disorders (Nofzinger & Keshavan, 2002). I will argue that it is an important source of neuropsychiatric symptomatology of PD. Although it is well known that a lack of sleep impairs arousal and attentional processes (Bonnet, 2000), recent advances in the study of sleep and cognition have revealed that both of the major mammalian sleep states [REM and non-REM (NREM) sleep] facilitate fundamental processes of neural plasticity and memory consolidation (Hobson, Pace-Schott, & Stickgold, 2000; Huber, Ghilardi, Massimini, & Tononi, 2004; Maquet, Smith, & Stickgold, 2003; Stickgold, 1998). Disruption of normal sleep processes, therefore, should disrupt memory and learning functions in addition to arousal and attentional functions. Disruption of these basic cognitive functions can lead to psychiatric disturbances (Nofzinger & Keshavan, 2002). There is now considerable evidence, for example, that disruption of sleep severely undermines normal functions of arousal, attention, learning, and memory (Dinges et al., 1997), thus impairing the ability to learn accurately, think, and act. Sleep deprivation, particularly REM sleep deprivation, also leads to mood dysfunction (Bonnet, 2000). Enhancement of REM intensity or duration is also associated with mood disorders of various kinds and to thinking/concentration problems as well. The inability to think clearly in the context of affective dysregulation can contribute to psychiatric disturbances.

Sleep appears to function, in part, to facilitate learning and memory (see collection of papers in Hairston & Knight, 2004; Hobson & Pace-Schott, 2002; Huber et al., 2004; Laureys et al., 2001; Maquet et al., 2003; Walker, Brakefield, Hobson, & Stickgold, 2003), though not all memory systems are equally affected or are affected in the same way or degree by sleep deprivation. Sleep-associated consolidation of information gathered during the wake state appears to depend on hippocampal–cortical interactions that occur during both NREM slow-wave sleep (SWS) and REM sleep and involve some sort of replay during REM sleep of learned associations acquired while awake (Buzsáki, 1996; Plihal & Born, 1997; Smith, 1995; Wilson & McNaughton, 1994). Wilson and McNaughton (1994), for example, showed that hippocampal cells that are active when rats learn a new maze are also active during subsequent sleep. Using positron emission tomography (PET) and other scanning techniques, similar effects (reactivation of brain sites activated during learning) have been reported in humans (Laureys et al., 2001). Stickgold, Hobson, Fosse, and Fosse (2001) have reported that learning a visual discrimination task was disrupted by selective deprivation of both REM and NREM sleep. Similarly, Plihal and Born (1997) have reported that learning of paired associates and mental rotation tasks, but not procedural memory tasks, is dependent on subsequent NREM (early sleep) rather than REM (late morning sleep) periods for their consolidation. Thus, whereas both sleep states appear to participate in learning and memory, their roles in consolidation of memories are postulated to be quite different but equally important. In short, sleep is crucial for learning and memory, and disruption of sleep impairs fundamental cognitive functions of attention, learning, and memory. Disruption of fundamental processes of arousal, attention, learning, and memory via disruption of sleep should, therefore, impact cognitive and affective functioning in PD.

How Might Sleep Disturbances Contribute to Mental Dysfunction in PD?

Recent neuroimaging studies of brain activation patterns during REM sleep demonstrate that the sites most activated in REM sleep are sites classically associated with emotional processing. These are the sites that I have associated with mediation of the minimal self. REM sleep, for example, is associated with extremely high activation levels in anterior cingulate, limbic, and amygdalar sites, as well as *deactivation* of dorsal prefrontal areas, parietal cortex, and posterior cingulate (Braun et al., 1997;

Hobson & Pace-Schott, 2002; Maquet & Franck, 1997; Maquet et al., 1996; Nofzinger, Mintun, Wiseman, Kupfer, & Moore, 1997). Given the evidence for a central role for the amygdala and the limbic system in mediating emotional states, particularly fearful and anxious states (Aggleton, 2000; Ledoux, 2000), this pattern of REM sleep–related brain activation implicates REM sleep states in emotional processing. Consistent with these imaging results, a recent review of studies of selective deprivation of REM sleep concluded that REM sleep deprivation heightens drive states in animals and perturbs emotional balance in humans leaving the sleep-deprived person "less interpersonally effective" (Bonnet, 2000). The well-documented association of sleep dysfunction, including reduced latency to first REM sleep period and an overall increase in REM duration in association with depression (Benca, 2000) supports the view that sleep processes are important for the regulation of mood states.

In summary, while the details of sleep-related cognitive and affective processing functions have yet to be worked out, there is now solid evidence that suggests that both REM and NREM sleep are required for normal memory and affective function and that disruption of these sleep states leads to significant affective and memory impairments in rats, in non-human primates, and in humans. I suggest, therefore, that sleep deficits of PD contribute to the cognitive, affective, and neuropsychiatric symptoms associated with PD.

Special Role of REM Sleep Disturbances in PD

REM sleep disturbances are, in fact, often associated with the onset of psychiatric symptomatology such as hallucinations (Arnulf et al., 2000; Goetz, Leurgans, Pappert, Raman, & Stemer, 2001), and affective disturbance (Starkstein, Preziosi, & Robinson, 1991) in affected PD patients. REM sleep, in particular, appears to play a role in production of psychiatric symptomatology of PD. Although REM sleep has long been known to be altered in depression (for reviews, see Armitage, 2007; Nutt, Wilson, & Paterson, 2008; Tsuno, Besset, & Ritchie, 2005), its role in production of symptomatology of depression of PD has only recently received attention. The repeatedly confirmed fact that both selective REM sleep and total sleep deprivation provides dramatic and immediate (though temporary) relief of both motor problems and depression for some people with PD (Demet, Chicz-Demet, Fallon, & Sokolski, 1999; Giedke & Schwarzler, 2002) supports the claim that REM sleep does indeed play some role in production of at least some depressive symptoms in some people with PD. REM sleep–related measures such as REM sleep density and REM dreams and nightmares are significant predictors of suicidal ideation in depressed individuals (Agargun et al., 1998; McNamara, 2008). REM-related indices of persons with posttraumatic stress disorder (PTSD) predict severity of PTSD (Germain & Nielsen, 2003). Indeed incorporation of trauma-related memories into REM dreams is one of the *Diagnostic and Statistical Manual of Mental Disorders*, 4th edition (DSM-IV; American Psychiatric Association, 2000) criteria for the disorder.

Burden of Sleep Dysfunction in PD

Numerous recent reviews of sleep problems in PD have emphasized that sleep problems in PD (a) are more frequent than previously suspected, (b) are underdiagnosed and undertreated, and (c) increase disability and caregiver burden when present (Happe & Berger, 2002; Happe, Ludemann, & Berger, 2002; Karlsen, Larsen, Tandberg, & Jorgensen, 1999; Larsen & Tandberg, 2001; Stacy, 2002). We (Wegelin, McNamara, Durso, Brown, & McLaren, 2005) recently confirmed the high prevalence of sleep disturbance in PD in midstage patients and found, in addition, that the sleep problems were significantly related to mood dysfunction in these patients. Other investigative teams (Boeve, Silber, Ferman, Lucas, & Parisi, 2001; Olson, Boeve, & Silber, 2000; Schenk, Bundlie, & Mahowald, 1996; Turner, 2002) have reported similar associations between sleep and cognitive and mood dysfunction in affected PD patients.

Although the exact prevalence of sleep problems early in the course of PD is unknown, up to 90% of patients develop sleep problems as the disease progresses, and approximately equal percentages of patients develop varying degrees of cognitive and mood dysfunction. In about half of these patients, the cognitive and mood disturbances become so severe as to require hospitalization or nursing home placement. It is therefore vitally important to identify predictors of cognitive and mood dysfunction in patients with PD so that early interventions can be developed to prevent or to ameliorate these conditions.

The Neuropathology of PD Affects Sleep Centers

As reviewed in earlier chapters, the primary pathology of PD involves loss of dopaminergic cells in the substantia nigra and in the ventral tegmental area (VTA; Agid, Javoy-Agid, & Ruberg, 1987). These two subcortical dopaminergic sites give rise to two projection systems important for arousal, motor, affective, and cognitive functioning. The nigrostriatal system, primarily implicated in motor functions, originates in the pars compacta of the substantia nigra and terminates in the striatum. The mesolimbic–cortical system contributes to cognitive and affective functioning. It originates in the VTA and terminates in the ventral striatum, limbic sites, amygdala, frontal lobes, and some other basal forebrain areas. DA levels in the ventral striatum, frontal lobes, and hippocampus are approximately 40% of normal (Javoy-Agid & Agid, 1980; Scatton, Javoy-Agid, Rouquier, Dubois, & Agid, 1983). The degree of nigrostriatal impairment correlates with degree of motor impairment, and VTA–mesocortical dopaminergic impairment correlates positively with the degree of affective and intellectual impairment (German, Manaye, Smith, Woodward, & Saper, 1989; Torack & Morris, 1988) in affected individuals.

Although these dopaminergic systems are major contributors to motor and cognitive dysfunction in PD, Lewy body degeneration, and Alzheimer-type changes have been noted in brain-stem nuclei (including the noradrenergic locus caeruleus and the serotonergic dorsal raphe nucleus—two sites implicated in sleep and arousal mechanisms), limbic structures, cholinergic forebrain structures, and in cerebral cortex (Emre, 2003; Jellinger, Seppi, Wenning, & Poewe, 2002). The cholinergic pathology in the basal forebrain structures and the Lewy body–type degeneration in limbic and in cerebral cortex are also likely contributors to sleep disorders, dementia of PD, and to affective dysfunction of PD.

Profile of Sleep Disturbances in PD

Sleep problems of varying degrees occur in up to 74% to 98% of patients with PD (Kumar, Bhatia, & Behari, 2002; Partinen, 1997). The patient with an early stage or midstage parkinsonian syndrome may present with complaints of insomnia, excessive daytime sleepiness, intense dreams, and abnormal movements at night. Laboratory [polysomnographic (PSG) and electroencephalographic (EEG)] studies of sleep in PD patients who are not depressed and not demented show decreases in sleep efficiency, as well as increases in sleep fragmentation with multiple night wakings (Aldrich, 2000).

Insomnia

Insomnia refers to the inability to get a good night's sleep. PD patients with insomnia lie awake at night, and when they finally fall asleep, they awaken a couple of hours later feeling unrefreshed. PSG and EEG studies of sleep in PD patients who are not depressed show decreases in deep sleep, too much light sleep (stage 2), as well as increases in sleep fragmentation and multiple night wakings. The motor problems of PD very likely contribute to insomnia. For some patients, it even becomes difficult to turn over in bed to get comfortable.

Excessive Daytime Sleepiness in PD

Excessive daytime sleepiness (EDS) is a common complaint of both early stage and midstage PD patients and may be related to reduction in sleep efficiencies and the increase in sleep fragmentation noted above. EDS is found in as many as 50% of PD patients and serious fatigue in about 60% of patients. Periodic limb movements, obstructive sleep apnea, and depression may also contribute to sleep maintenance problems and EDS. In addition, parkinsonian medications themselves may contribute to the excessive sleepiness. Frucht, Rogers, Greene, Gordon, and Fahn (1999) reported that use of the newer non-ergot DA agonists, pramipexole and ropinirole, was associated with sudden and irresistible "sleep attacks" during the day in some PD patients. But, Razmy, Lang, and Shapiro (2004) using the Multiple Sleep Latency Test (MSLT) to objectively measure EDS reported that patients treated with the newer non-ergot agonists did not differ from patients treated with the older ergotiline (bromocriptine or pergolide) agonists with respect to mean MSLT scores. The best predictor of pathologic daytime sleepiness was high LD dose or high dose equivalents of the other dopaminergic agents. In sum, the causes of EDS in PD patients remain unclear, but dopaminergic dose level is likely to be an important contributor.

In a study of midstage PD patients, we (Wegelin et al., 2005) found that that patients reported significantly greater levels of daytime sleepiness than those of age-matched controls and that this EDS was related primarily to anxiety levels (as measured by the Depression Anxiety and Stress Scales, or DASS; Lovibond & Lovibond, 1995) rather than to depression, stress, stage of disease, neuropsychological dysfunction, or to medication-related factors (see figure 9.1). Our multiple regression analyses of neuropsychological, mood, and medication-level correlates of EDS in patients with midstage PD revealed that anxiety levels were more strongly related to EDS than were neuropsychological dysfunction or dopaminergic dosing level.

Pal, Calne, Samii, and Fleming (1999) studied 40 nondemented patients with PD complaining of some form of sleep disturbance and 23 of their primary caregivers (all were spouses). They administered the Pittsburgh Sleep Quality Index, Zung's self-rating depression and anxiety scales, Parkinson's Impact Scale (PIMS; only for

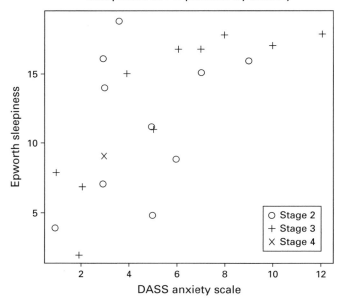

Figure 9.1
Epworth sleepiness score by DASS anxiety score for PD patients.

PD), and an additional sleep questionnaire. They found that 57.5% of patients complained of excessive daytime fatigue. Several component sleep scores correlated with anxiety scores, and subjects with global sleep scores greater than or equal to 10 (where 5 meant "problem sleep") had a higher mean anxiety index. There was no correlation between the degree of sleep dysfunction and the age, severity, duration of PD, or its drug treatment.

Although we are talking here only about two studies that have identified anxiety as important in EDS and fatigue in PD, the link may be an important one to document given the role that anxiety plays in the lives of persons at risk for PD and persons with PD themselves. If the link between EDS and self-reported anxiety proves to be causal, this finding could lead to a relatively straightforward treatment for EDS: treat the anxiety. If pathologic daytime sleepiness may sometimes put the life of the patient in danger (e.g., if the patient drives an automobile when sleepy), then developing effective treatments for pathologic EDS is an urgent necessity.

Sleep Disordered Breathing and Sleep Apnea in PD

Sleep apnea is one of the understudied, but vitally important, sleep disorders of PD. Apnea refers to episodes of cessation of breathing during sleep. Central sleep apnea refers to a problem in the brain-stem centers that control respiration. Obstructive sleep apnea refers to blockage in the breathing passages (nose, throat, etc.). Often, the blockage is excessive fat in the neck. Many people with sleep apnea are overweight. The patient with apnea very often snores quite loudly so that bed partners need to find they have to sleep in another room if they are to get any sleep themselves. When the patient with sleep apnea attempts to enter deep sleep, he stops breathing, and then this lack of oxygen prompts him to wake up briefly to get some air. The awakening may not be conscious as it is often very brief, but it may happen dozens of times each night so that the person's sleep is fragmented and filled only with light rather than deep restorative sleep. During the daytime, the individual feels overwhelming fatigue and a drive for sleep.

Periodic Limb Movement Disorder and Restless Legs Syndrome

Periodic limb movements during the night are quite common in the elderly, including PD patients. Restless legs syndrome (RLS), which is frequently associated with periodic limb movements, is frequently seen in the middle-aged population, in the elderly, and in PD. In both disorders, there is a sensation in the legs that causes the patient to move his or her extremities and may contribute to insomnia (Montplaisir, Nicolas, Godbout, & Walters, 2000). The PD patient with RLS often feels an irresistible urge to move the legs around during the night to get comfortable. Naturally, if you are moving your legs around at night, you are probably waking up more often and therefore are not getting a good night's sleep. This restless legs phenomenon may be one source of insomnia in PD.

REM Sleep Behavior Disorder

Although estimates vary dramatically, it appears that approximately 50% of PD patients have partial or complete loss of muscle atonia during REM sleep (Aldrich, 2000). This loss of the normal motoric inhibition of REM sleep may lead to physical enactment of REM dreams, many of which appear to be violent with the patient or his wife being attacked by intruders, and so forth, and the patient physically, and sometimes violently, reacting to the dreamed attack. This, of course, is dangerous both for the patient and his bed partner (patients and wives have been physically injured during an enactment episode).

The presence of RBD in a large proportion of PD patients supports the idea that REM sleep dysfunction is a major pathophysiologic source of psychiatric symptomatology in PD. There may be varying degrees of REM sleep disinhibition in the entire PD population, with RBD representing one end of the spectrum. It is instructive to examine the panoply of psychiatric phenomena associated with RBD as they may exist in the rest of the PD population but in muted form.

Hallucinations are common in RBD. I will say more about hallucinations in the larger PD population later. In the group of PD patients with RBD, hallucinations take on the following form: They almost always involve elaborate scenes of attack and aggression with the patient fighting back or attempting to escape the attack. Common hallucinatory behaviors of RBD include screaming, punching, grasping, kicking, and sometimes jumping out of the bed. The hallucinations are so real for the patients that they often injure themselves during an episode. Indeed, injuries are reported by more than 75% of patients (Schenck & Mahowald, 2002). The hallucinations appear to be directly driven by the REM sleep state as arousal from hallucinatory episodes is often accompanied by a dream recall that matches the observed behavior. Video-PSG monitoring reveals that hallucinatory episodes typically occur during REM sleep.

The dreams reported by patients with RBD may contain clues as to the genesis of hallucinatory states as well as delusions and other psychiatric symptoms of PD. This is because dreams of RBD patients turn out to be quite constant. All RBD patients, by and large, dream of the same themes. The most common dream theme reported by patients with RBD is that they are attacked by strangers or animals and they try to fight back in self-defense or attempt to flee (Schenck & Mahowald, 2002). Fear and anger are the most commonly reported emotions associated with the dreams, whereas aggression is the most constant theme.

Indeed, even very precise dream content studies show that the dreams of RBD patients are remarkably similar across different ages, sexes, and disease histories. It may be then that a common pathophysiologic process is producing the common dream content. That pathophysiologic process is REM sleep disinhibition.

One recent study has systematically assessed the dream content of RBD patients (Fantini, Corona, Clerici, & Ferini-Strambi, 2005). This study included 49 patients with PSG-confirmed RBD and 71 healthy controls. Dreams were elicited from participants and subjected to standardized dream content analyses. Fantini et al. (2005) found that compared with controls, patients with RBD reported a very high degree of aggression in their dreams. Sixty-six percent of RBD dreams and only 15% of control dreams had at least one episode of aggression. The characters involved in the aggression were largely males (96% males vs. 4% females) in the RBD group, whereas the sexes were almost equally represented in the control group (55% males vs. 45% females). Animal characters were more frequently present in RBD dreams than in control dreams (19% vs. 4%), but none of the patients with RBD had a "dream with at least one element of sexuality." By contrast, 9% of control participants had at least one dream with a sexual element in it. In short, the dreams of RBD patients display a remarkable consistency—they are filled with aggression, with the dreamer both on the receiving end of an aggression and acting as an aggressor himself. These RBD dreams are extraordinarily vivid and stand in marked contrast with the placid natures of the patients themselves during the daytime.

The Importance of Vivid Dreaming in RBD and in PD   To date, there are no studies that have examined potential relationships between dream content of RBD patients and the emergence of psychiatric disorder in PD patients, but I predict that the former will strongly predict the latter. Even in the absence of RBD, vivid dreams in PD are often the first sign that daytime behaviors will be affected. Sometimes vivid dreams are a prodromal symptom for daytime hallucinations. At other times, they may herald either an increase in or a decrease in daytime social aggressiveness. It may be that dreaming, in general, functions to modulate daytime mood, especially disposition to aggression. Notably, REM dreams appear to specialize in simulation of aggressive social interactions, whereas NREM dreams do the opposite—they simulate friendly interactions.

REM Sleep-Related Dreams Simulate Aggression   Using the standardized Hall/Van de Castle dream scoring scales (described under Methods; Domhoff, 1996), McNamara, McLaren, Smith, Brown, and Stickgold (2005) scored REM and NREM dreams and wake reports for number and variety of social interactions. We found that (1) social interactions were more likely to be depicted in dreams than in wake reports and (2) aggressive social interactions were more characteristic of REM than NREM dreams or wake reports. Dreamer-initiated friendliness was more characteristic of NREM dreams than REM dreams. It is important to note that dreamer-initiated aggressive interactions were *reduced to zero* in NREM dreams, and dreamer-initiated friendly interactions were twice as common in NREM as in REM dreams. It is, therefore, apparent that the lack of aggression in NREM dreams was not due simply to fewer social interactions occurring in NREM relative to REM dreams as friendly interactions in NREM dreams were more likely to be dreamer-initiated than in REM dreams (90% vs. 54%, respectively, $p < 0.05$).

These data were recently replicated using standard PSG and EEG sleep-staging techniques (McNamara et al., 2010). We awakened 64 healthy young volunteers from EEG-verified REM and NREM sleep states and then analyzed dream reports. As in our previous study with the nightcap technology, we found that in dreamer-involved aggressive interactions, the dreamer was the aggressor in 58% of REM dreams and in only 29% of NREM sleep-related dreams. In dreamer-involved friendly interactions, the dreamer was the befriender in 71% of NREM dreams and in only 42% of REM dreams. These data suggest that REM and NREM sleep may exhibit specializations in preparing the dreamer for aggressive versus friendly social interactions.

RBD and Vivid Dreams of Aggression May Predict Later Onset of PD   Varying degrees of RBD may be present for years before the motoric manifestations of PD develop. The emergence of vivid dreams filled with aggression may, in turn, constitute the first signs of a developing RBD process. In a large series of patients ($N = 93$) described by Olson et al. (2000), the nighttime dream-related *enactment behaviors* developed an average of 3 years before the motoric disorder (parkinsonism) in about half of those who had both conditions. Of those examined, between one third and one half of the RBD patients had PD, with a miscellaneous assortment of PD-related disorders (many involving synucleinopathies) accounting for the rest of the patients. In a later study, Onofrj et al. (2002) reported that of 80 consecutive patients with PD, 5 had RBD at baseline, 9 had developed RBD 3 years later, and 27 (34% of the original sample) had developed RBD at 8 years follow-up. The data of Onofrj et al. suggest that between one fifth and one third of PD patients will develop RBD over a 3-year period.

Sleep and Hallucinations in PD

Vivid dreams in PD often predict daytime hallucinations (Pappert, Goetz, Niederman, Raman, & Leurgans, 1999; Stavitsky et al., 2008). Many PD patients without overt RBD report episodes of hallucinations. Here, too, there is evidence that REM disinhibition is fueling the hallucinatory phenomena. Hallucinations are thought to be experienced by as many as 33% of PD patients during the course of their illness. They are generally thought to be a complication of dopaminergic pharmacotherapy and when present limit drug therapy for motor disability. They are, furthermore, a significant risk factor for nursing home placement (Goetz & Stebbins, 1993). Hallucinations in PD tend to occur in the visual rather than auditory modality and are frequently associated with vivid dreams. Notably, sleep disturbance is more common in hallucinators than in nonhallucinators (Pappert et al., 1999).

Sleep and Depression in PD

Chronic depression is seen in approximately 40% of PD patients, and major depression will be experienced by virtually all PD patients at some point in the course of the disease (Cummings, 1992). Although there can be little doubt that some portion of depressive illness is reactive, there is strong evidence to suggest that depression of PD is due to pathophysiologic processes of PD itself. Major depression in PD is unlike reactive forms of depression in that it is characterized by prominent anxiety and less proclivity toward self-punitive ideation. Depression of PD is more likely to occur in patients with right onset of the disease and, thus, with left-sided brain dysfunction. In patients with stroke, lesions of the left substantia nigra are more likely to produce depression than motor dysfunction. How can a lesion in the left substantia nigra produce depression? Because the substantia nigra is integrated into a circuit that ultimately impinges on prefrontal networks, anything that affects the substantia can also affect prefrontal function. Prefrontal dysfunction is known to occur in most forms of depression. A lesion in the left substantia nigra will reduce left external globus pallidus inhibition on the internal globus pallidus (due to loss of dopaminergic input to the striatum) and would lead to increased internal pallidal inhibition on thalamocortical activation of dorsolateral and medial frontal cortex.

REM sleep disinhibition leads to a similar deactivation of the DLPFC; therefore, REM sleep disinhibition in early PD could lead to both depression of PD and to executive cognitive deficits of PD. How so exactly? To explain it, it will be necessary to review briefly the known pathophysiology of depression and the physiology of REM sleep.

Brain Mechanisms of Depression

In the chapter on mood disorders of PD (chapter 10), I refer to Mayberg's model of the pathophysiology of depressive disorders (Mayberg et al., 1997, 1999). She presented a limbic–prefrontal interactional model of depression that consists of three neurofunctional "compartments" that account for differing clusters of depressive systems. Cognitive disturbances of depression are related to dysfunction in the dorsal compartment of the model, which includes the DLPFC, the dorsal anterior cingulate, and the posterior cingulate. Emotional, vegetative, and somatic symptoms of depression (affect, sleep, and appetite) are associated with disturbances of the ventral compartment, which consists of orbitofrontal, paralimbic cortical, subcortical, and brain-stem regions. If the dorsal system is damaged or inhibited by any physiologic dysfunction (e.g., disinhibited REM sleep in our scenario), then the ventral system would be released from regulatory constraints and would exhibit chronic overactivation. REM sleep is associated with downregulation of the dorsal PFC (dPFC), and thus, disinhibited REM sleep would chronically inhibit dPFC activity.

REM Sleep Normally Activates the Ventral System and Deactivates the Dorsal System

Brain activation patterns in REM sleep demonstrate high activation levels in limbic/amygdaloid sites and portions of mPFC but *hypoactivation* of DLPFC sites (Braun et al., 1997; Maquet et al., 1996, 2005; Nofzinger et al., 1997). This set of findings has been confirmed and extended by Nofzinger et al. among others Nofzinger et al. (1997, 2004) found that a consistent anterior paralimbic REM activation area that extends from the septal area and hypothalamus into ventral striatum, hippocampus, insula, ACC, orbitofrontal cortex, and SMA (Nofzinger et al., 1997, 2004). Reactivation of this midline and ventral anterior paralimbic area, as well as deactivation of dorsal prefrontal regions with the transition into REM sleep, has now been widely replicated (Braun et al., 1997; Maquet et al., 1996; Nofzinger et al., 1999, 2001, 2004; Pace-Schott, 2007; Smith et al., 1999; Wu, Buchsbaum, & Bunney, 2001; Wu et al., 1999). In short, REM normally activates the ventral system and deactivates the dorsal system in healthy people. Thus, it appears that each REM sleep episode is associated with a reproduction of key aspects of the neuroanatomy of depression and it is, therefore, not unreasonable to ask if REM sleep can negatively impact dorsal and ventral systems in such a way as to be depressogenic in PD patients.

REM Sleep Indices Are Enhanced in Depression

Reduced REM sleep latency and increased REM density and REM time (all signs of disinhibited REM sleep) are commonly observed in depressed patients (Kupfer & Foster, 1972; Tsuno et al., 2005). REM sleep deprivation can temporarily alleviate depressive symptoms (Giedke & Schwarzler, 2002; Vogel, Thurmond, Gibbons, Sloan, & Walker, 1975). Thus, signs of enhanced REM sleep pressure in some depressed patients may reflect a primary symptom of the disorder rather than a mechanism compensating for the affective disturbance (Gottesman & Gottesman, 2007; Van Moffaert, 1994).

Most antidepressant drugs reduce REM sleep (Winokur et al., 2001), and degree of REM suppression has been correlated with degree of symptomatic relief in responders (Giedke & Schwarzler, 2002; Vogel et al., 1975). REM sleep is associated with downregulation of biogenic amines, especially serotonin, and upregulation of acetylcholine. Whereas most antidepressants appear to suppress REM sleep globally by enhancing serotonergic activity, some agents do not have this effect. Nefazodone and bupropion do not globally suppress REM sleep (Winokur et al., 2001). Nevertheless, even these agents likely exert their antidepressant effects via their impact on the ventral and dorsal PFC systems. Nefazodone and bupropion, for example, either directly or indirectly enhance catecholaminergic activity in both the ventral *and dorsal* systems, thus reestablishing hierarchical regulatory control by the dPFC in these systems.

REM Sleep Deprivation

As mentioned above, REM sleep deprivation has an antidepressant effect and probably works by reestablishing hierarchical regulatory control by the dPFC over ventral system structures. Investigators using a variety of neuroimaging methods SPECT: Ebert, Feistel, & Barocka, 1991; Ebert, Feistel, Barocka, & Kaschka, 1994; Ebert, Feistel, Kaschka, Barocka, & Pirner, 1994; Volk et al., 1992, 1997; [18F]fluoro-deoxyglucose PET ([18F]FDG PET): Smith et al., 1999, 2002; Wu, Gillin, Buchsbaum, Hershey, & Johnson, 1992; Wu et al., 1999) have discovered that varying types and degrees of sleep deprivation have the effect of decreasing activation levels in ventral component structures and normalizing activation levels in dorsal system structures. Degree of decrease of activation levels in ventral component structures (as well as other structures like the basal ganglia), relative to pre–sleep deprivation baseline, predicts degree of antidepressant response to sleep deprivation therapy. For example, using [18F]FDG PET, Wu et al. (1999) studied the cerebral metabolic response to total sleep deprivation in 36 depressed patients and 26 healthy controls. At baseline, depressed patients who eventually responded to sleep deprivation showed elevated metabolism in the mPFC, ventral anterior cingulate, and posterior subcallosal gyrus. After sleep deprivation, activation levels declined in these ventral component structures, particularly the mPFC, and *increased* in the right lateral PFC in the sleep deprivation responders. Similarly, Wu et al. (2008) demonstrated decreased activation levels in ventral system structures and increased activation levels in DLPFC in six depressed subjects who had undergone and responded to one night of total sleep deprivation. Antidepressant effect (as measured by the Hamilton Scales) was correlated with changes in these brain activation levels/patterns. Similar effects are achieved with partial sleep deprivation procedures, though it is not yet clear whether REM sleep deprivation procedures are superior to NREM sleep deprivation or total sleep deprivation procedures (Giedke & Schwarzler, 2002; Gillin, Buchsbaum, Wu, Clark, & Bunney, 2001).

In short, REM sleep disinhibition should be considered a prime candidate source for depression, including depression of PD. Given the fact that REM sleep is also associated with deactivation of dorsal prefrontal networks, it may also be a source of prefrontal dysfunction and associated ECF deficits of PD.

Summary

Sleep problems of varying degrees and types occur in up to 74% to 98% of patients with PD (Kumar et al., 2002; Lees, Blackburn, & Campbell, 1988; Partinen, 1997). The patient with an early stage or midstage parkinsonian syndrome may present with complaints of insomnia, EDS, intense dreams, and abnormal movements at night. Laboratory (PSG and EEG) studies of sleep in PD patients who are not depressed and not demented show decreases in sleep efficiency, as well as increases in sleep fragmentation with multiple night wakings (Aldrich, 2000). There may also be intrusions of alpha activity into REM sleep in the early stages of PD (Wetter et al., 2001). By contrast, in normal aging, sleep problems involve a reduction in SWS duration and few if any abnormalities of REM sleep (Bliwise, 2000). Normal aging is also associated with increased numbers of arousals and a phase shift toward earlier bedtimes and early morning awakenings (Carskadon & Dement, 2000). As we have seen, some sleep problems may predict later PD by as much as a decade or more. Vivid dreams filled with aggression are also strong predictors of behavioral change as well.

Disturbances in sleep, with its related consequences for cognition and affect, cause hardships both for the patient and for the caregiver. Because of these hardships, and because of the lack of understanding and treatment options for the sleep disorders that contribute to them, we urgently need new approaches to the identification, analysis, and treatment of risk factors for these three classes of disorders seen in PD. Furthermore, an understanding of the causal relationships between these disorders may lead to better treatment and to better quality of life for PD patients. In particular, if sleep dysfunction contributes to the development of cognitive (e.g., dementia) and affective (e.g., depression) dysfunction in PD, then early and aggressive therapies to treat sleep disorders could delay the development of dementing illnesses and affective disorders in this population.

I recommend a large-scale prospective or longitudinal study of sleep changes in PD. Cognitive, sleep, and affective dysfunction are common in PD patients and independently predict disability and loss of independence, yet there has never been a prospective study of sleep, affect, and cognition in PD that assesses linkages of these three domains of functioning. Specifically, no study has yet examined the impact of sleep problems on daytime cognitive or affective functions. Identifying new factors that contribute to mental dysfunction in PD is critical to understanding causal factors of dementia and depression in PD and can lead to more effective therapies for PD patients. In addition, such a study may illuminate mechanisms of affective and cognitive impairment in normal aging and in many of the other age-related disorders that manifest such impairment. Specifically, data from such a study could result in a new avenue of approach to treating cognitive and affective dysfunction in PD. If sleep dysfunction contributes to neuropsychiatric disorders of PD, then early and aggressive pharmacologic and behavioral therapies to treat the sleep disorders may delay development of neuropsychiatric and dementing illnesses and of affective disorders such as depression and anxiety. Pharmacologic approaches that disturb sleep would likely be used less often, whereas therapies that enhance sleep efficiency would likely be increased if the understanding of sleep functions in PD were more widespread.

For example, the use of DA agonists prolongs the benefit of LD, but they can also be sedating. The latter effect may help with the sleep maintenance difficulty of PD. Pergolide, a DA agonist that has a D_1 receptor action, may cause some stimulation and a delayed sleep onset. However, the other DA agonists that exhibit a greater affinity for D_2 and D_3 receptors seem to be slightly sedating. With respect to the issue of sleep disturbance and depression in PD, current strategy relies heavily on serotonergic agents that are typically used to treat primary depression in otherwise healthy individuals. Some antidepressant agents have more pronounced effects on sleep architecture than others. They appear to "normalize" REM/NREM sleep architecture (Benca, 2000), and this normalization is associated with greater therapeutic effect. If further study of sleep functions in PD confirms a significant impact of sleep variables on cognitive and affect variables, then these types of antidepressant agents (i.e., those that normalize REM sleep) may be indicated even in early stages of PD.

If the reader has come with me this far, he or she will not be surprised at the predictions I offer concerning the origins, symptomatology, and nature of the mood disorders (anxiety and depression) that commonly occur in PD. I will also offer a brief review the symptom complex called apathy of PD. I review the symptoms of the major mood disorders of PD in this chapter and offer an explanatory model for those symptoms that derives from the larger theory of the agentic self system in PD that I have outlined in previous chapters. Hyperactivity within the amygdala is theorized to play a central role in mood disorders of PD.

Mood Disorder as a Dysfunction in the Agentic Self System

How can hyperactivity within the amygdala lead to such a wide variety of mood disorders? Depression is a very different experience than anxiety, for example, yet both, to some extent, derive from aberrant activity in the amygdala along with dysfunction in prefrontal systems. Apathy, in turn is different from both depression and anxiety. How, then, does aberrant activity in the amygdala give rise to varying forms of mood dysfunction, and what is the origin of apathy in PD? With respect to depression and anxiety, one possibility concerning their origins is that it depends on which potion of the amygdala is most affected by loss of inhibition from the DLPFC. Anxiety may result when the DLPFC and anterior PFC are impaired and the central nucleus of the amygdala (the output center for transmitting signals concerning danger) is disinhibited. If the central nucleus of the amygdala transmits message of danger, then the individual will become anxious, defensive, and harm avoidant. If that danger message is chronically transmitted then depression may result.

If the DLPFC is impaired in such a way that the basolateral nucleus of the amygdala is more hyperactive than the other nuclei of the amygdala, then these other intra-amygdalar nuclei may become silent or inhibited relative to activity in the basal nucleus. The basal nucleus sends excitatory afferents to a group of inter-calated cells in the amygdala that act as an inhibitory gate on cells in the major output center of the amygdala—the central nucleus If the cells of the basolateral nucleus become hyperactive (due to reduced regulatory control coming from the DLPFC and the orbitoprefrontal cortex), then efferents from the basolateral nucleus will activate the intercalated cells, which in turn will inhibit the central amygdala output cells in the central nucleus. If nothing is being outputted from the central nucleus then apathy may result. The loss of a signal from the amygdala may ultimately disinhibit downstream structures that the amygdala normally acti-vates. In short, if one turns off the frontal lobes, this will lead to overactivity in the basolateral nucleus in the amygdala. The overactivity in the basolateral nucleus will turn on the intercalated cells that then turn off the inhibitory signal emanat-ing from the central nucleus. The loss of the inhibitory signal coming from the central nucleus leads ultimately to the release of downstream sites from inhibition and the expression of aberrant mood and behavior. Emotional expression, for example, may be muted or dramatically diminished. Or emotional processing in general may become dysfunctional and emotions will not be able to be used to facilitate effective decisions.

Consider, for example, that the basolateral nucleus is known to send excitatory efferents to the ventral striatum, particularly the nucleus accumbens circuit (Sesack & Grace, 2010). Modulatory effects of basal nucleus signals on networks in the nucleus accumbens circuit (NAC) are complex and appear to affect the magnitude of DA release in support of high-level decision processes around motivational, reward, and goal-directed behaviors (Jones et al., 2010; Simmons, Brooks, & Neill, 2007). Nevertheless, pharmacologic silencing of the basolateral nucleus does not result in cessation of DA release in the NAC or VTA (Jones et al., 2010; Simmons et al., 2007). Instead, lack of input from the basolateral nucleus simply decreases the magnitude of DA release in the ventral striatum. That implies that what the signal from the basal nucleus usually does is to enhance the magnitude of DA release in response to rewarding stimuli. Presumably, the signal enhances phasic bursting of DA neurons in the NAC. Now, if the basal nucleus becomes hyperactive, it can no longer perform this modulatory role vis-à-vis the ventral striatum, and phasic signaling declines just as if the basal nucleus was silenced rather than hyper-active. These sorts of inverse-U properties (too much or too little stimulation creates problems) are common to all modulatory systems. Because they are designed not merely to turn on or off other systems but instead to alter the magnitude of existing responses, they require optimal dosing schedules. Too high or too low a dose at either end of the inverse U will have similar deleterious effects on target systems that can operate only with midrange doses (at the top of the inverse U).

Neurology of Depression in PD

What are the ultimate effects of overdosing of the ventral striatum? Phasic DA signaling declines, and thus the ability of the individual to experience reinforcing properties of rewarding stimuli also declines, resulting ultimately in depression. When the DLPFC and anterior PFC are impaired and the basolateral nucleus of the amygdala is released from top-down regulatory influences, the net effect is overexcitation (or overdosing) in the ventral striatum and thus downregulation of the ventral striatum. Given that the ventral striatum is crucial for prediction and processing of reward and goal-directed behaviors, the result is an amotivational state like apathy and an overall diminution in pleasure and subjective well-being. I will discuss the evidence for these claims later. But first I will provide a short review of the experimental evidence for emotional processing deficits in PD. These emotional recognition and production difficulties will help us to understand the ways in which patients with PD cope with the depressive or anxious pull of the disease process.

Emotional Processing in PD

PD can take a terrible toll on one emotionally. It can affect one's sense of self, one's hopes for the future, and all of one's relationships. Although it is true that the medications designed to treat PD have allowed persons with PD to lead relatively normal lives, at least at the beginning stages of the disease, they do not halt the progression of the disease. As the disease progresses, the medications may lose their effectiveness for some persons with PD. Some medications, furthermore, may have side effects that can affect one mentally and emotionally. Thus, persons with PD are faced with a chronic illness that each day limits their activities, may also force curtailment of income-producing work and career activities—and that impacts all of one's primary relationships. It would be surprising if PD patients experienced no anxiety or depression given these daunting circumstances. The person with PD faces the prospect of deteriorating physical and mental functioning, the loss of primary relationships, dependency on others for activities of daily living, and the necessity of having to remain in treatment until the end of his or her life. What is remarkable is how little mood dysfunction there is in PD. Although estimates vary wildly, only about half the PD population consistently reports clinically significant anxiety or depression. Of course, one can find studies that identify far higher rates of these mood disorders in various PD populations, but most systematic surveys of the best studies done on mood disorders among PD patients consistently report that about half of the people with PD report a mood problem at some point in the illness.

It seems to me that that is a surprising result given the challenges people with PD face. Not only are these people less depressed than one would expect, but they are also remarkably willing to cooperate in challenging experimental treatments that include aversive procedures, drugs with side effects, and so forth. I believe that people with PD have unusually strong, self-reliant personalities that predate the onset of the motor symptoms (see chapter 6 on personality changes in PD), and this unusually courageous, industrious, and intelligent personality type carries them through the long course of the disease with less mood dysfunction than might have been expected. An alternative to this "high intelligence" explanation for PD resistance to mood dysfunction is that the prefrontal and amygdalar dysfunction that goes with the disease confers some amount of protection against awareness of the illness' negative effects. But, this "denial of illness" explanation does not jibe with the fact that PD patients typically display full awareness of the challenges they face. What are some of those challenges?

Denial

Most persons with PD go through a period of denial of the diagnosis or of the real severity of the disease. This is a healthy reaction that allows the individual to take the time necessary to integrate into his emotional life what he has just been told. The cardiologist Thomas Graboys (whom I mentioned in a previous chapter) recounted the story of his denial of the PD diagnosis quite vividly (Graboys & Zheutlin, 2008). He tells of very close friends and colleagues trying to find gentle ways to tell him that his physical and mental powers were failing, but he, in return, just felt angry at these well-meaning friends. He tells the poignant story of running into the chairman of the department of neurology at a famous Boston Hospital who said to him (after witnessing his gait and posture, etc.), "Tom, who is taking care of your Parkinson's for you?" It took many other such encounters until he finally could no longer deny that he had PD. Once the diagnosis is accepted, further struggles often ensue. The main struggle that I have witnessed in the many patients I have encountered over my many years of working with them is the struggle to maintain some form of independence for as long as possible. All too often this struggle gets symbolized in the desperate need to hold on to one's driver's license for as long as possible. The struggle to maintain independence and control over one's life is one of the most salient emotional concerns of PD patients throughout the course of the illness. It is never fully resolved as most PD patients never give up the fight. Is this denial or courage and persistence?

Anger

Another intense emotional response that virtually all persons with PD struggle with is anger. Indeed, a better word is rage—rage and anger at the injustice and unfairness of the situation—not just for themselves but for their families and loved ones. Perhaps the greatest concern most PD patients have expressed to me over the years is not concern for their pain, discomfort, or their personal needs. Instead, it is the concern that they will become a burden on their families. Men who go from being the provider for the family to a dependent in the family find it particularly difficult to cope with the disease. More and more we are seeing younger people getting PD, and some of these young-onset patients have young children. Their challenge is to find the strength to cope with both the disease and the myriad challenges of raising young children. People with PD are angry that they have been dealt such a difficult hand. Thus, studies on the emotional responses of PD need to take this enduring anger and rage into account when interpreting the results of such studies. The old psychotherapists who dealt with PD patients in the era before LD thought that one of the distinguishing characteristics of the disease was a barely suppressed rage at the disease. These old psychotherapists helped patients to integrate the anger rather than to deny it or deflect it onto others. This was an important accomplishment as it helped relationships with caregivers, and caregivers are absolutely crucial sources of help for people with PD.

At some point, every person with PD has to come to accept the reality of the disease and the limitations it imposes on one's activities. The aim, however, is to find a way to accept the reality of the disease without letting the disease define the identity of the individual or to dictate what that individual can and cannot do. Remarkably, most people with PD find a way to accept the disease without letting it define who they are. Acceptance helps one to channel anger and grief at the losses incurred into more promising avenues of resistance such as exercise, information gathering, and the creation of new friendships and relationships within the PD community. By far, the greatest source of emotional turmoil in the life of a person with PD is his relationship with others. The most important of those relationships for most people with PD is the relationship with the spouse or with the primary caretaker. The PD patient has to constantly find a way to not let the relationship's emotional balance slip into one of overdependency on the caretaker.

I have only scratched the surface of the emotional challenges each person with PD grapples with on a daily basis. PD presents an enormous range of challenges for the affected individual and for his family. It is natural to feel some anxiety and depression—even severe depression in some cases. It is natural to go through periods of despair and to give in to gloomy outlooks concerning the disease. The disease has this relentless quality to it for most people. It keeps on taking and taking and taking. It never lets you rest. Despite the emotional toll the disease takes on the individual, the data on emotional problems of PD reveal a remarkable story of resilience and courage.

Deficits in Emotional Processing?

The available experimental data on emotional processing function in PD suggest that PD patients have little difficulty reading emotions in the faces of others or in experiencing the normal range of emotions everyone feels in daily life. In our clinical experience, emotional changes of PD in midstages of the disease involve social withdrawal, lack of interest, reduced initiative in pursuing social interactions, and inability to express emotions in the face or in speech fully (due to motor problems).

Notably, persons with PD may instead find it difficult to perform higher-order or more complex emotional feats than simple experiencing of feeling or emotion. Telling a lie, for example, is an emotional accomplishment because it needs to be done without expressing emotional stress in the voice or face. Abe et al. (2009) have shown that persons with PD find it more difficult than healthy people to tell lies. When persons with PD show difficulty in telling white lies, they demonstrate less metabolic activity in the PFC than do healthy people when they are telling white lies. Apparently, you need a certain level of DA activity in the PFC to tell a convincing white lie, and because persons with PD find it more difficult to reach that level of DA activity in the PFC, they also find it more difficult to lie.

Telling a white lie or a big lie requires an agentic self system that is in possession of powerful executive control processes. These executive control processes have to suppress emotional activity, control facial and gestural displays, and maintain a strategic and manipulative stance toward others while the lie is being "told." This set of behaviors is all under the control of the agentic self, and thus lying can be considered a function of the agentic self. There are occasions when lying is so important the agentic self has to be kept in the dark about it. These are the cases that require the person to be self-deceived or to believe the lies he is telling others. Given the enormous amount of compartmentalization that must occur for this sort of self-deception to occur, I doubt that persons with PD could do it for long periods of time. In contrast, we have records of politicians with PD who functioned well as politicians right up to the end. I know of no studies of self-deception in PD.

Anxiety in PD

Anxiety and panic are estimated to occur in 40% of patients with PD. Again, it seems to me, this is a remarkably low figure given the problems PD patients face on a daily basis. The anxiety disorders of PD include social phobia, panic disorder, and unclassifiable forms of anxiety. The psychoanalysts who treated patients with PD back in the pre-LD era noticed that there was a higher incidence of claustrophobia among PD patients than in other clinical populations. I know of no controlled studies of this disorder in the PD population. Notably, when PD patients experience panic attacks, it is often during the off phase (off LD), and the anxiety can be relieved by administration of LD. The fact that anxiety disorders are ubiquitous among people with PD suggests that it is a defining feature of the illness. As I mentioned in the chapter on personality changes of PD, anxiety is the one constant feature of the PD personality. It appears long before the motor symptoms appear and persists long into the illness. Bower et al. (2010) collated data on 6,822 healthy subjects who were followed over four decades as part of a longitudinal Mayo Clinic study on personality and aging. The investigators found that an anxious personality profile documented at the beginning of the study (decades ago) was associated with an increased risk of developing PD. A depressive profile was *not* related to PD onset. Several other case-control or cohort studies (reviewed in Savica et al., 2010) have suggested that anxiety may be one of the earliest manifestations of PD even when analyses are restricted to 20 or more years before PD onset. Anxiety rarely appears alone in PD. It is often associated with cognitive impairment or with depression. I suggested above that anxiety in all populations including PD may result when the DLPFC and anterior PFC are impaired and the central nucleus of the amygdala (the output center for transmitting signals concerning danger) is disinhibited. An overactive amygdala yields a constant background mood of impending doom or dread and generalized fear. One solution might be to reinstate top-down prefrontal (PFC) regulatory controls over the amygdala.

The reactivation of the PFC can occur pharmacologically and via use of cognitive behavioral strategies such as cognitive-restructuring of issues that worry the patient, responding in writing to vague fears, graded exposure to phobic fears, practice in problem solving skills, and the like.

Depression in PD

PD is associated with a two- to four-fold increase in the risk for developing major depressive disorder (MDD) relative to other similarly disabling conditions. In about one half of the cases, the depression precedes the onset of motor symptoms in PD (Santamaria, Tolosa, & Valles, 1986). The fact that both anxiety and depression precede motor manifestations of disease by many years suggests to me that the initial pathology in the disease involves the prefrontal–subcortical/limbic loops that I have linked with the agentic self system rather than isolated nuclei in the brain stem as the Braak staging system suggests.

In any case, depression occurs in approximately 40% of PD patients. Once again, I find this statistic a remarkably low incidence given the ravages the disease inflicts upon its victims. I attribute the low rates of depression to the unusually high intelligence levels found among people with PD. The greater intelligence allows the patients to find more ways of coping with the illness than is the case in other chronic medical diseases. But, admittedly, I have no data to support this conjecture.

Depression Symptomatology in PD

The motor symptoms of PD sometimes mimic symptoms of depression. In major depression, as in PD, you see decreased activity or "poverty of movement," reduced speech output, psychomotor slowing (bradyphrenia), and a lack of motor fluency and initiative. Something like the PD "masked face" is sometimes also seen in major depression. There is a strange lack of emotional expression in the face. In the case of PD, this is due to depleted DA activation in facial musculature. In depression, its causes are unknown, but it is correlated with anhedonia and lack of feeling more generally. The bradykinesia or slowed movement in PD finds its counterpart in the lethargic movements seen in depressives. The loss of fundamental drives like eating, sex, and sleep is common to both disorders as well. What is different about the depression of PD (in comparison with MDD that occurs in other populations) is that it often involves anxiety (an anxious depression) but not guilt or self-blame. There may be suicidal ideation, but relative to MDD, there is a low suicide rate. In both MDD and PD depression, however, there are problems in ECFs like attention, concentration, resistance to interference, working memory, and the like. Another symptom that is very often comorbid with the depression of PD is apathy. Apathy involves a loss of motivation or initiative without loss of the ability to experience pleasure. The latter, anhedonia, is often a part of the picture of major depression. Apathy may occur either as a separate syndrome (12% of PD cases) or as a comorbid disorder with depression (30% of cases).

Keeping in mind these differences concerning the depression of PD versus MDD that occurs in other populations, we can now turn to consider the symptomatology and neurology of MDD as it occurs in both PD and in non-PD populations.

Major Depressive Disorder

MDD (American Psychiatric Association, 2000) is associated with a range of symptom clusters including the hallmark persistent sad, anxious, or "empty" feelings. Cognitive distortions of depression feature a barrage of negative self-appraisals that lead to feelings of hopelessness and/or pessimism, guilt, worthlessness, and/or thoughts of suicide, or even suicide attempts. There is often a variety of other cognitive distortions besides the major distortion regarding self-worth. These other cognitive distortions involve difficulty with concentration, planning, or making decisions (executive dysfunction). Memory, too, is affected with negative and painful memories favored in recall, in acquisition, and in consolidation processes. In addition, dreams become intensely unpleasant experiences with elevated levels of what used to be called *masochistic content* or scenes of aggression by unknown strangers against the dreamer/self (McNamara, 2008). Nightmares become more frequent occurrences in the dream life of the depressed individual and predict suicidal ideation (Agargun, Kara, & Solmaz, 2007).

Pathophysiology of Depression

Neurochemical Contributions to Depression in PD Depression in PD can be due to dysfunction in both the dopaminergic and serotonergic systems. There is degeneration of 5-hydroxytryptamine (5-HT; serotonin) producing cells in the raphe nucleus. The density of the midbrain serotonin transporter receptors is decreased in PD. There is a reduction in levels of the serotonin metabolite 5-hydroxyindole acetic acid (5-HIAA) in the cerebrospinal fluid of PD patients with depression. In addition, the degeneration of dopaminergic neurons in the VTA leads to a loss of phasic signaling in reward centers of the brain. Both dopaminergic and serotonergic agents can relieve some depressive symptoms in some PD patients.

This neurochemical pathology surely contributes to depressive symptomatology of PD, but the fundamental problem seems to be aberrant activation and deactivation patterns in corticolimbic loops that mediate what I have been calling the agentic self and minimal self systems.

Prefrontal–Limbic Loops in Depression Mayberg and colleagues (1997, 1999) presented a limbic–prefrontal interactional model of depression that consists of three neurofunctional "compartments" that account for differing clusters of depressive systems. Mayberg and colleagues' limbic–cortical model has informed many neurocognitive investigations of depression and is very close to what I proposed above regarding (basolateral nucleus) amygdalar–prefrontal interactions in depression. In Mayberg and colleagues' model, as I understand it, cognitive disturbances of depression are related to dysfunction in the dorsal compartment of the model, which includes the DLPFC and dorsal anterior cingulate and posterior cingulate. Emotional, vegetative, and somatic symptoms of depression (affect, sleep, and appetite) are associated with disturbances of the ventral compartment, which consists of orbitofrontal, paralimbic cortical, subcortical, and brain-stem regions. The rostral compartment (the rostral anterior cingulate cortex), corresponding with Brodmann area 24, has connections to both the dorsal and ventral compartments and may serve an important regulatory role in the overall network.

Prefrontal cortical systems are known to be organized in a hierarchical manner with the DLPFC exerting top-down regulatory control over ventromedial and orbitofrontal systems and functions (for reviews, see Botvinick, 2008; Fuster, 2008). If the dorsal system is damaged or inhibited by any physiologic dysfunction (e.g., due to PD), then the ventral system would be released from regulatory constraints and would exhibit chronic overactivation.

Consistent with the regulatory role of the dorsal system over paralimbic and other PFC circuits and functions, and consistent with Mayberg and colleagues' limbic–cortical model of depression, resting-state PET and SPECT studies in patients with unipolar depression have most consistently found *decreased* function in the DLPFC (e.g., Baxter et al., 1989; Drevets et al., 1992, 1997; Mayberg, 1994) and *increased* activation in ventral system structures (Drevets et al., 1997; Liotta et al., 2000). Once the dorsal system is impaired, the systems it regulates are released from top-down inhibitory control, and *increases* in activation of ventral system structures occur in depressed patients. Such increases in activity in depressed patients have been documented via rCMRglc and rCBF studies in ventrolateral, ventromedial, orbitofrontal cortex and subgenual prefrontal cortex, amygdala, and insular cortex (Drevets et al., 1997; Liotta et al., 2000).

Consistent with a causative role of these brain systems in production of depressive symptomatology, pretreatment abnormalities found in prefrontal and limbic–paralimbic areas in depressed patients appear to normalize with recovery from depression (Brody et al., 1999; Drevets et al., 2002; Goodwin et al., 1993; Kennedy et al., 2001; Mayberg et al., 2000; Sheline et al., 2001). This involves a normalization of frontal hypoactivity in the dorsal compartment and a decrease of activation levels in the ventral compartment.

Both lesion (Koenigs et al., 2008) and neuroimaging (e.g., Davidson, 2002; Drevets, 2007; Mayberg et al., 1999; Nofzinger, 2008) studies suggest that the pathogenesis of MDD involves abnormally high levels of activity in paralimbic structures and ventromedial prefrontal cortex (vmPFC) and abnormally low levels of activity in the DLPFC. The person with depression, therefore, cannot effectively recruit the DLPFC to regulate paralimbic and vmPFC-related negative emotional activity via reappraisal/suppression strategies (e.g., Ochsner et al., 2004). Attention in the field has therefore turned to the question of why paralimbic/vmPFC structures are chronically overactivated and DLPFC structures underactivated in MDD.

Drevets (2007) argued that a *visceromotor* circuit was crucial for understanding MDD. It consists of the dorsomedial/dorsal anterolateral prefrontal cortex (e.g., Brodmann area 9), the mid and posterior cingulate cortex, a region in the anterior superior temporal gyrus and sulcus, and the entorhinal and posterior parahippocampal cortex. This system is similar to the PFC–limbic loop that I argued supported the minimal self. Drevet's visceromotor circuit displays dense interconnectivity with limbic structures and visceral control structures (hypothalamus and periaqueductal gray) and closely resembles the "default system" network that has been defined in human functional imaging studies as a system that displays baseline activation values in the resting state. It seems to "appear" whenever the individual is just sitting and being aware of self.

A wide array of pharmacological, neurosurgical, and deep brain stimulation treatments for MDD appear to work by suppressing pathologic activity within visceromotor network structures such as the subgenual anterior cingulate cortex, amygdala, and ventral striatum (Drevets & Price, 2005), thus confirming the role of these structures in MDD.

Depression and Cognitive Deficit in PD

Depression in PD appears to be linked with deficits in an array of ECFs. Depression in PD increases the risk of developing dementia in later stages of the disease.

Treatments for Depression in PD

Several of the standard antidepressants appear to work for depression in PD, but there have been surprisingly few double-blind, placebo-controlled studies of antidepressant agents for depression in PD. A potentially fatal complication may result from the combination of a selective serotonin reuptake inhibitor (SSRI) with the MAO-B inhibitor selegiline. This combination can cause a very rapid rise in central nervous system serotonin levels and, in severe cases, death. The DA agonists have relatively weak antidepressant properties. LD appears to improve mood in most patients, but once depression develops, LD seems not to alleviate its symptoms.

A relatively new treatment for depression in PD is use of repetitive transcranial magnetic stimulation (rTMS). In this treatment, magnetic impulses are transmitted to particular regions of the brain by applying magnetic coils over those regions of the brain. rTMS has been shown to be effective in the treatment of MDD in non-PD patients with few or no side effects. It is not clear how long the positive effects last, however, and there have been few double-blind, placebo-controlled trials of the treatment. Open-label trials demonstrate that rTMS has antidepressant effects in PD patients with depression, but again, these are open-label trials, and it is known that PD patients display very strong placebo effects. Cognitive behavioral therapy and interpersonal psychotherapy, either alone or in combination with pharmacotherapy, are effective treatments for some symptoms of MDD and of depression in PD. There is new evidence that one form of treatment has both strong antidepressant effects and positive effects on both motor and cognitive symptoms of PD. That treatment is aerobic exercise. Studies in both humans and animals have shown that physical exercise, particularly aerobic exercise like walking, running, swimming, bicycling, and so forth, promotes the release of neurotrophic factors—these are chemicals that bathe brain cells in nutrients that allow the brain cells to grow and make connections with other brain cells. In addition, aerobic exercise increases the amount of blood and oxygen to the brain, thus enhancing virtually all brain functions. Studies of exercise treatment programs with PD (Goodwin, Richards, Taylor, Taylor, & Campbell, 2008) have shown pretty conclusively that exercise improves physical functioning, strength, balance, and gait speed. There are exercise programs that have been specifically designed for persons with PD, and these appear to have antidepressant effects as well.

Apathy in PD

If the essence of the PD deficit is a profound impairment in the system of agentic self with a resultant overactivation in the system of the minimal self, then we would expect to see a global reduction in initiative and in energetic pursuit of goals (even in the absence of depression). This overall reduction in the capacity to initiate goal pursuit and in novelty seeking, more generally, would be related to deficits in ECFs because it would be due, from my point of view, to an impairment in some component part of the agentic self.

Impairment of different components of the agentic self yield varying forms of disorder. If the impairment is at the level of valuation or identification of values or of rank ordering those values in order of importance, then an emotionally based apathy may be the result. If the deficit is at the level of choosing one of those values to pursue (i.e., a deficit of decision making along with ECF deficit), then impulsivity may be the result. If the deficit is at the level of generation or formulation of plans and goals to pursue chosen values, then a cognitive form of apathy may result. If the deficit involves inability to implement plans to obtain rewards, when pursuing a goal or reward a form of depression may emerge, and so forth. Cognitive and emotional forms of apathy nevertheless share some fundamental features (see table 10.1). I suggest that commonalities among forms of apathy are due to the fact that the impairment of the agentic self is at the root of apathy.

So, what aspect of the agentic self is impaired in apathy of PD? There is not enough data in the literature to yet decide the issue, and I have not conducted

Table 10.1
Diagnostic criteria for apathy according to Starkstein et al. (2009)

A. Lack of motivation relative to the patient's previous level of functioning or the standards of his or her age and culture.
B. Presence, while with lack of motivation, of at least one symptom belonging to each of the following three domains:

Diminished goal-directed behavior
1. Lack of effort or energy to perform everyday activities.
2. Dependency on prompts from others to structure everyday activities.

Diminished goal-directed cognition
3. Lack of interest in learning new things or in new experiences.
4. Lack of concern about one's personal problems.

Diminished concomitants of goal-directed behavior
5. Unchanging or flat affect.
6. Lack of emotional response to positive or negative events.
7. The symptoms of apathy cause clinically significant distress or impairment in social, occupational, or other important areas of functioning.
8. The symptoms are not due to diminished level of consciousness or to the direct physiologic effects of a substance.

studies on the disorder myself. What little data exist and pilot data I and my colleague, Erica Harris, have gathered suggests that when apathy occurs in PD without comorbid depression or dementia, the main cause of the apathy appears to be cognitive deficit at the level of generation of plans to pursue goals. That suggests that the key sites of dysfunction are in the DLPFC and in frontopolar cortex, Brodmann area 10. Most other investigators of apathy in PD tend to assume the causative lesion or site of dysfunction is in the mesial PFC near the supplementary motor cortex or in the ACC. These sites are certainly involved in the production of apathy as well, but the available data link the apathy of PD to ECF deficits rather than to depression or to motor initiation problems. Although apathy in PD certainly does often occur with depression, one can get apathy in PD without depression. The problem is not an emotional one or one of motor initiation (at least an initiation problem that is above and beyond what normally occurs in PD). It is, instead, a cognitive problem. The apathy of PD appears to be linked most consistently to ECF deficits, most specifically, to goal formulation, planning, and monitoring of goal pursuit, and so forth.

Clinical Phenomenology of Apathy in PD
Various authors have estimated the frequency of "apathy plus" syndromes in PD (i.e., when apathy occurs in tandem with depression or dementia) is anywhere between 17% and 70% of patients. When apathy occurs alone, the frequencies range from 12% to 39%. Starkstein et al. (2009) reported that 52 (32%) of the 164 PD patients they studied met diagnostic criteria for apathy. Eighty-three percent of these patients had "apathy plus." Forty PD patients had neither depression nor dementia, and only five of these had apathy. Nevertheless, those five cases indicate clearly that one can get apathy without also having depression or dementia. We need to see apathy as more than just a subtype of depression. It is its own disorder with its own neurobiologic and cognitive mechanisms that are different from those of depression or dementia.

Levy–Dubois Subtypes
On the basis of a review of the literature on the anatomy of apathy, Levy and Dubois (2006) suggested three major subtypes of apathy. Their cognitive-affective subtype most closely corresponds with the apathy syndrome seen in PD in my opinion. Cognitive-affective apathy involves lesions of the DLPFC and the dorsal caudate nucleus, the internal portion of the globus pallidus, the lateral substantia nigra pars reticulata, and the anterior thalamic nuclei (Levy & Dubois, 2006). Patients with PD

who suffer from this type of apathy perform poorly on tests of ECFs and planning including the Stroop Color-Word Interference Test, categorical verbal fluency, the Tower of London, and the Wisconsin Card Sort Test (Levy & Dubois, 2006). Emotional-affective apathy is linked with dysfunction in the orbital-medial PFC and the limbic regions of the basal ganglia including the ventral striatum and ventral pallidum. Autoactivation deficit is most often associated with lesions in the medial PFC and limbic areas of the basal ganglia, particularly in the internal portion of the globus pallidus (Levy & Dubois, 2006).

Measurement of Apathy

Several types of scales have been developed to measure various subtypes of apathy (van Reekum, Stuss, & Ostrander, 2005). The four most commonly used apathy scales are the Apathy Evaluation Scale (AES; Marin, 1996), which is not validated for use in PD; a 14-item version of the Apathy Scale (a brief form of the AES), which has been validated for use in PD; the Lille Apathy Rating Scale (LARS; Sockeel et al., 2006), which has been used with PD patients; and the Apathy Inventory (AI; Robert et al., 2002). It is assumed that these four scales measure the same thing, but I have not seen any studies that report correlations between scores on these scales.

Starkstein, Mayberg, Preziosi, et al. (1992) assessed apathy in a group of 50 PD patients. Twelve percent of the sample exhibited apathy without depression. Levy et al. (1998) found that apathy [as measured by the Neuropsychiatric Inventory (NPI)] was correlated with Mini Mental State Exam (MMSE) scores but not depression. Similarly, Aarsland et al. (1999) found that 4.3% of patients with untreated PD had apathy and no depression. Pluck and Brown (2002) found that apathy scores in PD were correlated with executive function tests. Kirsch-Darrow et al. (2006) found that about one third of their sample had apathy without depression. Dujardin et al. (2007, 2009) found that performance on a battery of executive function tests reliably distinguished demented versus nondemented PD patients. Pedersen et al. (2009) found that patients with apathy at a baseline test session were significantly more likely to have dementia at follow-up 4 years later. Oguru et al. (2010) found that 15% of a sample of PD patients had apathy without depression or dementia, and apathy scores were correlated with poor cognitive performance. Pedersen et al. (2010) administered the NPI to a group of de novo PD patients 25 of who had apathy without depression. Apathy was significantly associated with attention and executive deficits. Note that in virtually none of these studies (except Pedersen et al., 2010) was apathy significantly related to motor severity or stage of disease.

Summary

The basic theory I have been arguing for in this book concerning mental dysfunction in PD is that the agentic self is only weakly activated in people at risk for PD and even more weakly activated in people with actual PD. This weak activation of the agentic self system has significant consequences for all of the neuropsychiatric disorders of PD, especially for the mood disorders of PD. Because the agentic self system regulates and inhibits the set of neural structures associated with what I have been calling the minimal self, then it follows that those structures (that mediate the minimal self) will become disinhibited and unregulated when there is a weakly activated agentic self. In addition, when the agentic self is for one reason or another almost totally suppressed, then apathy results. The neural structures that mediate the agentic self are the DLPFC, the rostral or anterior or frontopolar PFC, portions of the hippocampus, the ACC, and some nuclei in the neostriatum, the basal ganglia, and the cerebellum. The key structures for the agentic self, however, are the DLPFC (understood to include supplementary, premotor, and motor areas), the frontopolar PFC, and the ACC. The neural structures that mediate the minimal self are the limbic system, the amygdala, portions of the hippocampus, the ventral striatum (like the NAC), and the vmPFC/medial portions of the orbitofrontal cortex (OFC). When the agentic self system is impaired, these latter sets of structures become disinhibited in varying degrees depending on the anatomic distribution of the lesions the PD degenerative process happens to follow in the affected individual. I suggest that mood disorders of various kinds result when the mesolimbic/mesocortical dopaminergic systems are impaired, resulting in reduced activation levels in the DLPFC. The reduced activation levels of the DLPFC leads to a reduction in inhibitory powers of the DLPFC. The weak inhibitory signals emanating from DLPFC efferents to target sites in the limbic region leads to hyperactivity in the amygdala and the orbitofrontal cortex. This amygdalar hyperactivity is the ultimate cause of mood disorders in my opinion.

As the neurodegenerative process that underlies PD progresses, risk for developing psychotic ideation and a dementing illness increase significantly. At least 75% of PD patients who survive for more than 10 years will develop some form of PD dementia (PDD; Aarsland & Kurz, 2010), but there is huge variation with some individuals not developing dementia at all, some developing a relatively mild form of dementia, and some not developing dementia until very late in the disease. The mean time from onset of PD to dementia is approximately 10 years. The strongest predictors for development of early dementia in PD are old age, postural and gait disturbances, and impairment in *frontal* ECFs (Janvin et al. 2006; Kulisevsky & Pagonabarraga, 2010; Marder, 2010). Because the ECFs are treated in this book as part of the agentic self system, in our terms, severe impairment in the agentic self system increases risk for later dementia in PD. Thus, if the agentic self system can be "exercised" so that ECFs and speech acts are frequently practiced and used in everyday life, then it may be that risk for dementia can be diminished or forestalled. It is known, for example, that intelligence and educational attainment reduce the risk for senile dementia in non-PD populations, and it seems reasonable to assume that this is the case for people with PD as well. Of course, no one knows for sure if dementia is an inevitable part of the PD course as it is impossible to follow all PD patients throughout their lives, but I have seen a very large number of persons with PD who die at a ripe old age having never become demented. Nevertheless, a majority of people with PD develop some form of dementia in later stages of the disease. It and psychosis represent major neuropsychiatric disorders of PD. What happens to the agentic self in PDD? To answer that question, we will first need to survey the clinical phenomenology of PDD itself.

Clinical Phenomenology and Pathophysiology of Dementia in PD

Most people understand dementia of any type to involve impairment in virtually all cognitive domains: perception, language, thinking, belief, memory, emotion, visuo-spatial functions, and so forth. With respect to the dementia seen in late stages of PD, the Movement Disorder Society (MDS) task force in 2007 (Emre et al., 2007) suggested the following specific diagnostic criteria for dementia of PD (PDD):

Preexisting PD should be determined by the UK Parkinson's Disease Society Brain Bank criteria (Gibb & Lees, 1988). There must be must be a decline in cognitive performance from a premorbid performance level and affect two or more of the following four cognitive domains: attention, executive function, visuoconstructive ability, and memory. The cognitive impairment, finally, must be observed to impair daily function in social or occupational domains. As is the case with any other diagnosis, one also has to rule out competing or alternative diagnoses that might account for the cognitive decline. There are two forms of dementia that can often look like PDD: dementia with Lewy bodies (DLB) and Alzheimer's disease dementia (ADD). DLB is diagnosed when dementia either precedes or occurs within 1 year of onset of PD motor symptoms and when other core symptoms such as attentional fluctuations and visual hallucinations are present (Emre et al., 2007; McKeith et al., 2005).

From a practical and clinical point of view, PDD can be considered to be present when (1) the patient has PD as established by the UK/Queen's Square Brain Bank criteria (Hughes et al., 1992), (2) onset of motor symptoms was at least 1 year prior to onset of dementia, (3) scores on the Mini Mental Status Examination (MMSE) (Folstein, Folstein, & McHugh, 1975) decline to < 26, and (4) activities of daily living are impaired. The requirement (by the MDS task force) for impairment in attention, executive function, or working memory is particularly interesting as these functions are part of the agentic self. These executive functions are less affected by ADD than by PDD. Instead, in ADD, memory systems are more impaired than the executive system (Brønnick, Emre, Lane, Tekin, & Aarsland, 2007). PDD, in my view, afflicts the agentic self, whereas ADD afflicts the minimal self.

PDD is associated with a variety of cognitive deficits including deficits in the domains of executive, attentional, and visuospatial function. Executive dysfunction is the most consistently reported deficit. Even when memory is impaired in PDD, the impairment usually involves strategic search through memory fields rather than loss of memory information, per se. Although the bulk of the patients with PDD exhibit this profile of severe dysfunction in executive systems, some investigators have claimed that a smaller group of PDD patients have significant memory problems. Thus, there may be three types of PDD: a dysexecutive, amnestic, and mixed type (Janvin et al., 2006; Lewis, Slabosz, Robbins, Barker, Owen, 2005). The dysexecutive type is the most common. The amnestic type involves a marked problem in memory recall, but again, this is usually due to strategic search problems rather than recognition memory (memories are not gone; they are just more difficult to retrieve in PDD). Nevertheless, PDD of the amnestic type is sufficiently different from PDD of the dysexecutive type. Keep in mind that PDD presents itself to us in variable ways. The prominence of the impairment of systems of the agentic self in PD and PDD should not blind us to clinical heterogeneity of PD.

Depression, Apathy, and PDD

While depression most often precedes PDD, it can be a prominent symptom of PDD as well. When it occurs as part of PDD, it mimics motor symptoms of PD. Psychomotor retardation looks like bradykinesia and masked facies looks like loss of emotion, and so forth. Fatigue and sleep problems also occur in both depression and PDD. These symptoms are also found in apathy. Apathy is a loss of initiative, verve, energy, and drive. Approximately 60% of PD patients report significant amounts of apathy (Pedersen et al., 2009) when measured by the Neuropsychiatric Inventory (Cummings, 1997). Again, apathy is seen in PDD and in depression. Because apathy can occur without depression or dementia after frontal lobe lesions, it may be that both apathy and depression of PDD are due to prefrontal dysfunction.

Dopaminergic Contributions to PDD

One source of prefrontal dysfunction in PDD is the loss of dopaminergic innervation to PFC in PD itself. Both nigrostriatal and ventral tegmental area (VTA) DA efferents innervate portions of PFC. The ventrolateral portion of the substantia nigra innervates the putamen and is the site of greatest damage in PD. Medioventral and dorsal areas of the substantia nigra, however, connect to the caudate, which in turn sends efferents to PFC. Nobili et al. (2010) used single photon emission tomography with [^{123}I]ioflupane-CIT, a marker that binds to presynaptic DA transporter proteins, to study potential associations between DA activity in the nigrostriatal tract and ECF performance in volunteers. They found a positive correlation between caudate uptake of ioflupane-CIT in both hemispheres and performance on tests of ECF. The efferents sent from the VTA up to PFC sites are also important for ECF. Rinne et al. (2000) used [^{18}F]fluorodopa PET to study dopaminergic activity in the PFC of PD patients and found it to be significantly reduced relative to levels in controls. The greater the radioactive fluorodopa uptake in the frontal lobes (indicative of more intact direct mesocortical dopaminergic innervation), the better was the performance on various ECF tasks. Cools, Stefanova, Barker, Robins, & Owen (2002) reported LD-induced increases in cerebral blood flow were significantly diminished in right DLPFC when participants were challenged with a planning task. Mattay et al. (2002) used functional magnetic resonance imaging (fMRI) to study brain activity patterns during a working memory task of PD patients both on and off LD. Increased activity in frontal lobes during the working memory task was most evident only when patients were off LD, suggesting that there was an attempt to recruit more frontal cortex to perform a task that is normally handled by more restricted regions of the PFC.

The Special Role of Norepinephrine in ECF Deficit in PD

Though not usually considered as a candidate in the explanation of cognitive deficits in PD, there is evidence that the role of norepinephrine (NE) is crucial. Postmortem studies of cortical NE and MHPG consistently report decrements of these indices in PD patients with cognitive dysfunction. The locus caeruleus suffers severe cell loss in PD ranging from 21% to 93%, with an average of 63%. Locus ceruleus (LC) cell loss correlates significantly with cognitive symptoms in PD, being more severe in patients with dementia than in those without dementia. LC damage results in severe loss of cortical and limbic NE innervation with a 40% to 78% decrease in NE, its metabolites, and related enzymes in PD. These changes are most marked in patients with significant cognitive deficits. There are significantly decreased numbers of LC neurons *in dopa-unresponsive PD patients* relative to dopa-responsive patients. In clinical studies, Stern, Mayeux, and Cote (1984) found significant correlations between NE metabolite levels in PD patients and performance on reaction time tasks and continuous performance tasks that measure attention and vigilance.

Riekkinen, Kejonen, Jakala, Soininen, and Riekkinen (1998) reported strong correlations between measures of NE levels and attentional cognitive performance in PD. Bedard et al. (1998) reported significant improvements on measures of attention and distractibility in a series of PD patients who were given the alpha-1 noradrenergic agonist naphtoxazine. Lemke (2002) reported significant improvement on self-rated and objectively rated scores on a number of depression inventories in 16 PD patients with moderate to severe depression after 4 weeks of treatment with reboxetine, an NE reuptake inhibitor. In short, there is now clear evidence that NE dysfunction plays a role in the production of cognitive and mood deficits of PD.

Cholinergic Contributions to PDD

The neurobiology of PDD may be linked with dysfunction in forebrain systems that use acetylcholine as a neuromodulator. It may be that dysfunction in cholinergic systems either causes or contributes to dementia of PD; it certainly is a contributing factor in the case of AD (Whitehouse, Hedreen, White, & Price, 1983). Thus, either PDD patients may have a form of AD or cholinergic dysfunction may simply be a contributing factor to PDD. In one study, PET was used to image both dopaminergic activity with [^{18}F]fluorodopa and cholinergic activity using N-[^{11}C]-methyl-4-piperidyl acetate (MP4A) in PD patients with and without dementia and in age-matched healthy controls (Hilker et al., 2005). In patients with dementia, Hilker et al found that cholinergic MP4A global cortical binding showed significant reductions of 29% versus controls, whereas patients without dementia demonstrated moderate reductions of 10.7% compared with controls. Two other studies used similar PET techniques and reported similar results in PDD (Bohnen et al., 2003; Shimada et al., 2009).

Although there is clear cholinergic pathology in PDD, as mentioned above, PDD exhibits a very different cognitive profile than that of AD. PDD patients evidence greater degrees of ECF dysfunction and lesser memory abnormalities than those of AD patients (Aarsland, Litvan, Galasko, Wentzel-Larsen, & Larsen, 2003; Litvan, Mohr, Williams, Gomez, & Chase, 1991; Noe et al., 2004; Pillon, Deweer, Agid, & Dubois, 1993). I summarized this distinction by suggesting that PDD is an affliction of the agentic self, and AD is an affliction of the minimal self. Both AD and PDD patients evidence abnormalities in visuospatial skills. The language disorders of PDD and AD differ as well. In AD, there is initially a naming deficit and then fluent paraphasias and often a fluent aphasia. In PDD, a naming deficit may or may not be present, but there is a deficit in speech act comprehension (Holtgraves & McNamara, 2010a).

That cholinergic dysfunction must play some role in PDD is supported by some emerging neuropharmacologic treatment studies. To date, however, only one large-scale placebo-controlled study has examined the use of an acetylcholinesterase inhibitor in PDD. Emre et al. (2004) randomly assigned 541 patients with mild or moderate PDD to placebo or to 3–12 mg daily oral doses of rivastigmine. In the 410 patients who completed the study, there was statistically significant improvement in validated measures of cognitive performance as well as in activities of daily living. Performance by patients assigned to the placebo condition actually declined on some measures. In a follow-up study (Poewe et al., 2006) that allowed the patients assigned originally to placebo to cross over to the treatment arm of the study, patients who crossed over to the active drug showed gains similar to those of the drug treatment group in the original study.

Psychosis in PD

Psychotic symptoms refer to the development of hallucinations (seeing, hearing, smelling, etc., things that are not real) and/or delusions (believing things that are not real). When persons with PD develop psychotic symptoms, families and caregivers are much more likely to attempt to place the patient in a nursing home. Delusions appear to be less common than hallucinations in PD, and when present, they often co-occur with hallucinations and cognitive impairment (Kulisevsky, Pagonabarraga, Pascual-Sedano, Garcia-Sanchez, & Gironell, 2008; Marsh et al., 2004). Psychotic symptoms are very distressing to families and caregivers because the individual actively hallucinating or in a delusional state is very often a danger to himself or herself and sometimes a danger to others. For example, we (McNamara & Durso, 1991) described an elderly patient with PD who had developed a fixed delusion that his wife was cheating on him. This is known as *Othello syndrome* after Shakespeare's tragic character, Othello, who kills his wife in the mistaken belief that she had been unfaithful to him. Our patient pointed to the most bizarre features (such as flashing lights in the yard that were supposedly the headlights of the car of the wife's lover, stains on the bedsheets, etc.) as evidence to prove his wife's infidelity. The wife's advanced age, her stay-at-home schedule, the family, and every other piece of reliable evidence we could gather pointed to the wife's innocence. Yet, nothing could shake the patient's delusional belief system … until he was withdrawn from the anti-parkinsonian medication he was on at the time.

Psychosis is, in fact, rare until patients with PD are put on anti-parkinsonian medications. Drug-induced psychosis in PD ranges from 6% in early PD to 40% in advanced stages of PD. The DA agonists are more likely to cause psychotic symptoms than LD, presumably because they act predominately on limbic sites whereas LD acts predominately on neostriatal/PFC sites. Nevertheless, anti-parkinsonian medications seem not to be the main culprits in this story because many PD patients with hallucinations are not on higher doses of these medications than those of patients without hallucinations. Instead, the risk factors point to sleep disorders (particularly vivid dreaming), cognitive deficit, depression, and advanced stage of the disease.

Visual hallucinations are reported in up to 74% of later-stage patients (Hely, Reid, Adena, Halliday, & Morris, 2008). This is an interesting phenomenon from the point of view of the neurobiology of PD because visual hallucinations are not as common in the equally devastating neurodegenerative disorder of AD despite the fact that brain pathology is typically more widespread in midstage AD than in midstage PD. In fact, visual hallucinations are much more common in PD than auditory, olfactory, or tactile hallucinations. Visual hallucinations in PD, furthermore, are not the fleeting shapes and colors of popular lore but instead are more typically complex, well-formed composite images of objects, people, and animals. The fact that the hallucinations are complex wholes suggests that their source involves changes in cortical sites or at least recruits those sites. Available data suggest that the patients most likely to develop these complex visual hallucinations are those with a history of vivid dreams and sleep disorders. Notably, many (about one third) PD patients experience hallucinations but are aware that they are doing so. This intact awareness keeps them out of the psychotic spectrum. When awareness/insight recedes and patients believe that the hallucinations are real, it becomes psychosis.

Mania

About 10% of persons with PD who are treated with dopaminergic agents will experience an episode of mania. In such an episode, the patient experiences a sense of euphoria, agitation, restlessness, and sometimes delusional beliefs. Episodes of mania are more likely when the patient has been given an anticholinergic in addition to dopaminergic agents. Mania and hypersexuality have been reported to occur after some forms of surgical treatment including implantation of a stimulator in the brain designed to stimulate the subthalamic nucleus. These manic episodes and hypersexuality can last up to several months.

Pathophysiology of PDD and Psychosis in PDD

Taken together, the above briefly reviewed clinical evidence concerning the mental symptoms of PDD and psychosis in PD, as well as the available neurobiologic evidence, all suggest that something more than PFC dysfunction has to contribute to the PDD clinical picture. Dementia, depression, apathy, hallucinations, and mania cannot all result from an impairment in the agentic self system, although that impairment must be considered core to the process that leads to PDD. Once the agentic self system declines, the risk for progression to PDD is higher, and we have seen that PDD is characterized by greater ECF deficits than that in AD. Nevertheless, the traditional view concerning the direct pathophysiologic causes of PDD lies in impairment in a series of neuroanatomic circuits, or loops, running between the

Table 11.1
Prefrontal–subcortical circuits

Motor	Cognitive	Motivation	Will/Affect
Motor circuit • Supplementary Premotor and motor cortex • Putamen • Globus Pallidus (ventrolateral) • Thalamus (VA and MD)	Dorsolateral circuit • DLPFC • Caudate (dorsolateral) • Globus pallidus (dorsomedial) • Thalamus (VA and MD)	Orbital circuit • Lateral Orbitofrontal cortex • Caudate (ventromedial) • Globus pallidus (dorsomedial) • Thalamus (VA and MD)	Cingulate circuit • Anterior Cingulate cortex • Nucleus accumbens • Globus pallidus (rostrolateral) • Thalamus (MD)

VA, ventral anterior; MD, mediodorsal.

basal ganglia and selected sites in the frontal lobes. I want to conclude this chapter by summarizing the traditional account of the pathophysiology of PDD because the account makes sense and helps us to understand why depression, apathy, and ECF impairment are core components of PDD. These frontal–basal ganglia loops are thought to contribute to the regulation of motor, motivational, and mental functions in PD. Although details of the specializations of each of the putative functional loops are problematic, the basic functional scheme seems clear enough (see table 11.1). The motor circuit, for example, modulates cortical output necessary for voluntary movement. When it is impaired, voluntary movement is impaired. The general functional scheme is this: Output from the motor (or motivational or cognitive or affective, etc.) circuit is directed through the internal segment of the globus pallidus (GPi) and the substantia nigra pars reticulata (SNr). This inhibitory output modulates the thalamocortical pathway itself and suppresses its actions (e.g., movement or thought depending on the circuit involved). To initiate movement, signals from the cerebral cortex are processed through the basal ganglia–thalamocortical motor circuit and return to the same area via a feedback pathway. When supplementary motor areas in the frontal lobes are released from subcortical inhibition, voluntary movement may occur. Similarly, a *cognitive circuit* runs between the thalamus, globus pallidus, the dorsal caudate nucleus, and thence to the DLPFC. The *motivational circuit* involves the ventromedial nucleus of the caudate and the lateral orbital frontal cortex, and finally, the limbic/emotional circuit involves the nucleus accumbens and the ACC. Impairment of each of these specialized circuits in PD may partially contribute to characteristic types of mental dysfunction in PD with impairment of the dorsolateral prefrontal loop accounting for deficits in ECFs; impairment of the orbitofrontal loop contributing to apathy and related neurobehavioral signs; and impairment in the limbic/cingulate circuit contributing to depression in PD. When all of these circuits are impaired to a significant degree, the result is PDD.

Two pathways exist within each basal ganglia–prefrontal circuit: a direct and an indirect pathway. In the direct pathway, outflow from the striatum directly inhibits GPi and SNr (i.e., the inhibitory modulating switch for the circuit itself). The indirect pathway comprises inhibitory connections between the striatum and the external segment of the globus pallidus (GPe) and the GPe and the subthalamic nucleus (STN). The STN exerts an excitatory influence on the GPi and SNr. The GPi/SNr sends inhibitory output to the ventral lateral nucleus of the thalamus. Striatal neurons containing D_1 receptors constitute the direct pathway and project to the GPi/SNr. Striatal neurons containing D_2 receptors are part of the indirect pathway and project to the GPe.

To influence both motor and mental clinical symptoms of the disease, various points in both the direct and indirect pathways have been targeted with pharmacologic, deep brain stimulation, and surgical techniques. These targeted interventions are thought to work by altering inhibitory/excitatory balances along the direct and indirect pathways as well as along the basal ganglia–prefrontal loops.

Dementia and psychosis may occur when all of these PFC–subcortical loops are affected by the disease. The dorsal PFC circuit is the first to go and weakens the agentic self. Then the orbitofrontal–limbic circuit is released from inhibition thus resulting in mood dysfunction. The brain-stem pathology associated with the disease and the hyperactive limbic loop leads to sleep dysfunction as well. The combination of all these abnormalities contributes to the distinctive dementia and psychoses seen in PD.

Impulse Control Disorders in Parkinson's Disease

An impulse control disorder (ICD) occurs when a patient loses control of his impulses around food, sex, money, gambling, and the like. What are the anatomic correlates of ICDs in PD and how does the agentic self fit into the picture of causal factors for ICDs in PD?

Here is one potential explanation of the anatomic correlates of ICDs in PD: The agentic self system is in mutual inhibitory balance with the minimal self system. Anatomically, when the dorsal PFC–basal ganglia loop is impaired, the ventral and orbitofrontal (OF)–limbic loop is disinhibited. Because the latter mediates fundamental drives of sex, food, and aggression, impulses associated with these drives are to varying degrees released from regulatory controls. When this situation occurs, the risk for developing ICDs increases significantly. These ICDs may involve compulsive gambling, hypersexuality, compulsive eating or spending, and the development of peculiar special interests such as special hobbies (Wolters, van der Werf, & van den Heuvel, 2008). ICDs can be devastating for PD patients and their families. Aside from the shame associated with ICDs, families can lose all their savings in one bout of compulsive gambling; hypersexuality can lead to criminal behaviors and divorce. It is clear that we need a better understanding of ICDs in PD.

Typically, in the case of persons at risk for PD, there is an imbalance in the dorsal versus ventral systems such that the dominant emotion is one of anxiety. The executive system is weak relative to the impulses it was designed to regulate. According to one reading of the Freudian tradition, when the executive system or ego is weakened but not overwhelmed by the impulsive system (the id), the response is anxiety and a generalized defensive reaction involving rigid adherence to moralistic norms, avoidance of harm and risk, low novelty seeking, cautiousness, and so forth. This latter constellation of traits is embodied in the structure of the superego, but as readers of this book will immediately recognize, this "superego" is none other than the premorbid personality profile of people at risk for PD. In short, a weakened agentic self system leads to an effort to strengthen it despite a disinhibited minimal self/impulsive system pressuring the agentic system. This effort to strengthen the executive control system (or *reaction formation*) results in the personality profile of PD, at least according to one reading of the psychoanalytic tradition on PD. In reality, of course, the individual is dealing with chronically low dopaminergic activity levels. The personality traits of low novelty seeking and high harm avoidance are simply the result of the reduced ability of phasic DA to suppress fear and anxiety and reinforce risky choices. There is no reason to exclude the psychodynamic description of this personality stance as long as we maintain a healthy skepticism concerning imputations of elaborate, hidden, and nefarious motives of individuals who exhibit the profile.

By the time the individual is diagnosed with PD, DA levels in subcortical–PFC loops are quite low. The agentic self system is starved for DA and it is correspondingly weakened. But, because DA levels in the VTA–PFC loops are also relatively low, the limbic–PFC loop is also weakened, and neither system has the upper hand. Administration of LD tends to slightly favor the agentic self system, but some individuals are also put on dopaminergic agonists; most of these agents decisively favor the limbic–PFC loop. At that point, the minimal self overwhelms the agentic system and the individual becomes more impulsive.

DA agonists were introduced as an adjunctive treatment for motor symptoms of PD in the 1980s but were not widely available until the mid-1990s. Subsequent studies of effects of these drugs in PD have consistently reported an association between initiation of treatment with DA agonists and development of ICDs. Aside from the intrinsic clinical importance of treating ICDs when they emerge, their emergence after initiation of agonist therapy underlines the neurobiology of agentic versus impulsive self systems in PD. If the addition of dopaminergic stimulation within the limbic–PFC loop can produce ICDs, then dopaminergic activity within the limbic–PFC loop must be key for the impulsive minimal self. When that stimulation occurs in the context of a weakened agentic self, the self system that normally inhibits impulsivity, then the risk for ICDs is enhanced.

As discussed in previous chapters of this book, patients with PD typically exhibit mild to severe deficits on tests of ECFs, and these deficits are linked, in turn, to decision-making biases. Performance of PD patients on the Iowa Gambling Task (IGT; Bechara et al., 1994) is in fact similar to that of compulsive gamblers and to persons who compulsively use addictive substances. PD patients off medication tend to be better at learning to avoid choices that lead to negative outcomes than they are at learning from positive outcomes. When patients are put on DA agonists, however, this bias in decision making is reversed. Positive reinforcers become stronger than the wish to avoid losses.

DA Agonists and ICDs in PD

There is a strong association between initiation of DA agonist therapy in PD and ICDs (Wolters et al., 2008). ICDs only rarely occur (1% of patients) when the patient is on LD alone. When patients are given DA agonist therapy, about 15% will develop ICDs. In one study of cases of compulsive gambling in PD, 98% of them were on an agonist of one kind or another. It is not clear whether ICDs are dose dependent (i.e., whether they are more likely to emerge after administration of higher doses of DA agonists). Certainly, some patients develop ICDs on low doses of DA agonists and to some extent the effects depend on the particular drug.

For example, pramipexole exhibits high affinity for the DA D_3 receptor subtype. It is 10 times more potent at the D_3 than at the D_2 receptor. Because the D_3 receptor is expressed mainly in limbic and OF sites (whereas the D_2 receptor is prevalent in both limbic/OF and dorsal PFC sites), pramipexole may be particularly liable to promote ICDs. Pergolide is equipotent at D_2 and D_3 receptors, and bromocriptine is 10 times more potent at the D_2 than at the D_3 receptor. The affinities of pergolide and cabergoline for the D_3 receptor are comparable with that of pramipexole.

One additional factor that may facilitate development of ICDs and other compulsive behaviors is pulsatile dopaminergic activity. This sort of dopaminergic activity can be promoted when patients are given high potency, short-acting medications such as LD and subcutaneous apomorphine injections. Apomorphine is usually given to treat severe off states as physicians are aware of problems associated with promotion of pulsatile DA activity.

Prevalence of ICDs in PD

Voon et al. (2006) reported a 6.1% lifetime prevalence of ICDs (pathologic gambling, hypersexuality, compulsive shopping, or a combination) in PD patients, but this estimate is acknowledged to be inaccurately low as it was based on self-report.

In PD patients, ICDs and compulsive use of dopaminergic medications (the *dopamine dysregulation syndrome*, or DDS) are associated with younger age and the male sex. Younger patients are prone to developing dyskinesia and motor fluctuations, and DA agonists are prescribed to delay these complications. In PD, individuals with ICDs and DDS have higher rates of other axis I psychopathology, including depressive symptoms, psychosis, and high alcohol intake.

Clinical Phenomenology of ICDs in PD

According to the DSM-IV (American Psychiatric Association, 2000), ICDs are characterized by a "failure to resist an impulse, drive, or temptation to perform an act that is harmful to the person or to others." ICDs described in PD include pathologic gambling, hypersexuality, compulsive buying, compulsive eating, kleptomania, impulsive–aggressive disorder, and trichotillomania.

Pathologic Gambling

Compulsive gambling is characterized by a preoccupation with gambling; the loss of ever increasing amounts of money; unsuccessful attempts to control the problem; deception or covering up the extent of the problem; loss of work time; and harm to the individuals' primary relationships. Most compulsive gamblers, including PD patients, get hooked on things like the slot machine that very occasionally reinforces the risky behavior just when it is about to be extinguished. In addition, gambling on the Internet is becoming an increasingly problematic behavior for both PD and non-PD gamblers.

Sexual Disorders

When someone is preoccupied with sex for weeks, sometimes months on end, and when they let other parts of their lives suffer in pursuit of sex, then a problem with hypersexuality may be developing. If excessive use of pornography exists, if there is compulsive masturbation, if there are extramarital affairs, if there is a seeking-out of prostitutes, then hypersexuality may be present. If there is criminal behavior involved such as exhibitionism, or various paraphilias, sexual disorder exists (Fernandez & Durso, 1998). The emergence of hypersexuality and sexual disorder in PD is particularly dramatic because so many patients report loss of libido or problems with sexual function prior to treatment with agonists. Though numbers are hard to come by as there are very few controlled studies on this issue, it appears that at least 68% of newly diagnosed persons with PD report some problems with some aspect of sexual activity. These problems with sexual activity involve everything from impaired performance to decreased desire for sex.

Problems with sexual function in PD can be caused by several factors including low DA levels in the brain, aging, decreased ability to move, medication types and dosages, autonomic nervous system (ANS) dysfunction, and emotional issues such as depression and anxiety. There may also be lower levels of testosterone in some men with PD. The ANS controls many of those bodily functions that need to happen automatically and outside of our voluntary control such as the heartbeat, blood pressure, blood flow changes to meet a challenge, some aspects of breathing, and so forth. The ANS supports several facets of sexual performance from erections in men to lubrication and pelvic thrusting in women to orgasm in both men and women. ANS dysfunction is all too often part of the picture in PD, and thus ANS dysfunction may contribute to sexual problems in PD. Last, but not least, emotional problems associated with PD can also contribute to sexual dysfunction. Depression and anxiety can drain the pleasure out of virtually all activities including sex. Some medications that are used to treat depression (such as citalopram, fluoxetine, fluvomine, paroxetine, and sertraline) sometimes have side-effects in some people that result in reduced interest in sex.

There have been very few studies that examine the impact of PD on sexual functioning in women with PD. What little evidence that exists suggests that women with PD often experience a decline in sexual desire and a reduced ability to experience orgasm during sex. Sex can be uncomfortable due to lack of lubrication and desire. For women with PD who have experienced menopause, the decline in sexual interest may be due to both menopause and to PD.

Given all these potential sources of problems with sexual function, it is dramatic when a person with PD begins to develop hypersexuality. As mentioned above, this usually occurs when the patient is put on a DA agonist.

Compulsive Eating
For patients with this ICD, eating may occur in binges triggered by stressors. Often, binge eating occurs in the evening or in the middle of the night. Just as in the case of hypersexuality, the pattern of compulsive eating (and resultant weight gain) is in stark contrast to the usual weight loss that occurs in most persons with PD.

Compulsive Spending
Just as in the case of compulsive gambling, compulsive spending may be so extreme as to put the family savings in jeopardy.

Punding
When animals are given large amounts of drugs that stimulate catecholaminergic activity, they engage in repetitive motor behaviors, usually behaviors that are related

to appetitive drives like searching for food or mating opportunities. When human beings are given large amounts of catecholaminergics, they, too, engage in repetitive motor stereotypies, but the repetitive behaviors often have an individualistic shape to them. When, for example, a hobby becomes an obsessional interest and hobby-related activities begin to impinge on work and family time to such an extent that losses are incurred, then time spent on that hobby might be called *punding*. Typical examples of punding include repeatedly cleaning the house, collecting or sorting objects, tinkering with or dismantling household equipment or gadgets, and so forth. What is particularly interesting is that these behaviors emerge after administration of catecholaminergic agents, and when the patient is challenged about them he may get irritable and angry. Like compulsive eating, the repetitive activity often occurs overnight. Punders withdraw into themselves and are absorbed by the activity that has captured their attention and interest.

Dopamine Dysregulation Syndrome

Given that dopaminergic medications have reinforcing or rewarding properties, it should not be surprising that they sometimes can be used compulsively in order to achieve a "high." When patients use medications compulsively to such an extent that they incur losses in other areas of their lives and drug-induced side-effects are ignored, then the patient may be using the drug compulsively and dangerously. Patients with DDS often identify aversive "off"-period symptomatology as the reason for their compulsive medication use. The off period is certainly very often associated with very unpleasant effects such as depression, anxiety, and panic attacks, so it is no wonder that patients want to avoid this state.

The Variety of ICDs Experienced in PD Patients

Patients with PD treated with agonists testify to the central role DA plays in iden-tification of rewards, values, and the learning process more generally. When the limbic–OF loop becomes hyperactivated in the context of a weakened agentic self with executive function deficits, then ICDs may emerge. Most often, adjustments in dose of the agonist in question will reduce ICD manifestations, but the ideal treat-ment would be to strengthen the agentic self system. I will return to the issue of strengthening the agentic self in chapter 13.

13   Rehabilitation of the Agentic Self

Up to this point in the book, I have described an array of neuropsychiatric disorders that are sometimes seen in PD. However, I do not want to leave the reader with the impression that PD is nothing but a catalogue of deficits. Instead, one of the benefits of looking at PD from the point of view of the agentic self is that we can see that it is a person, an individual, who copes with an array of challenges including functional deficits. The individual is not a syndrome. The person, not the syndrome, lives in the face of and despite these deficits. When we focus on the agentic self, or the acting person, new opportunities for treatment and rehabilitation open up.

Rehabilitation Is Possible Only for a Person, Not a Syndrome

When we treat the person rather than the disorder, the disorder is tamed and made to serve the person. If we neglect the person, the disorder will dictate to the person. If we neglect the person, the disorder will define who the person is. To live, and to flourish, despite the disease, the person has to find a way to prevent the disorder from defining who he or she is and what he or she can do with his or her life. Only a person can find a way to live through an incurable disorder.

Ben-Yishay et al. (1985) have offered a model of the ways in which rehabilitation involves "ego-identity" change. Their holistic approach to rehabilitation of brain-injured persons inspired much of the early work on the role of the self in living through chronic effects of brain injury. Fotopoulou (2008) suggests that understanding confabulations as attempts by the brain-injured person to preserve self-concept and to facilitate ongoing identity formation can help us find better ways to deal with confabulations than just ignoring them. If one knows that the function of these confabulations is self-preservation and self-enhancement, one can better channel the patient's efforts in this direction by providing more healthy opportunities for self-enhancement than confabulation. Naylor and Clare (2008) report that AD patients with a more positive and definite sense of self were found to display poorer awareness of their memory function and a greater impairment of autobiographical memory during the midlife period. But, this poor awareness of the extent of their memory impairments actually meant that they functioned better and could likely maintain independence for a longer period of time than patients with a weaker sense of self and greater awareness of deficits. Cooper-Evans, Alderman, Knight, and Oddy (2008) found that sense of self was, not surprisingly, negatively impacted by brain injury. A higher level of self-esteem was related to reduced self-awareness and poorer cognitive function. Gracey et al. (2008) attempted to investigate determinants of the all-important sense of self of brain-injured persons in a group therapy context. They elicited bipolar constructs of self through structured small-group discussions in a holistic rehabilitation setting. They found that sense of self after acquired brain injury is constructed on the fly through daily subjective experiences associated with social and practical activities. That means that the sense of self might be strengthened by including daily activities designed to do just that. It is a remarkable fact that no rehabilitation program is comprehensively designed to use all methods available to strengthen the sense of self after brain injury or disease. Instead, "skills" of one kind or another are most often targeted for practice and instruction. For example, most people with brain disorders enter a standard rehabilitation program that can be called the Standard Social Skills Rehabilitation Training (SSSRT) program. SSSRT is composed of comprehensive training designed to improve daily coping skills, optimize medication adherence, and increase social and occupational functioning. Social interaction skills are practiced through group interactions, feedback, role-plays, and homework exercises. Groups are typically run by rehabilitation professionals such as speech therapists or occupational therapists.

But, how can a brain-injured person acquire these sorts of social skills if his sense of self is lost or submerged or weakened? First, we need to strengthen the self—the agentic self, in particular—and then that agentic self can help regulate attention, memory, and all of the other cognitive systems in such a way as to be able to learn. Cloute, Mitchell, and Yates (2008) used discourse analytic techniques to analyze interviews, conversation, and social interactions of patients with traumatic brain injury (TBI) and a significant other. They confirmed that instead of strengthening the sense of self in these patients, most interactions—even in a rehabilitative setting—have the effect of weakening the sense of self because patients are treated as passive interlocutors with nothing to contribute to the interaction. If we developed rehabilitation programs that were specifically designed to strengthen the agentic self, this sort of treatment of patients would be much less likely.

Existing Rehabilitation Approaches Directed at the Self

There are some initial stabs at developing treatment approaches that strengthen the agentic self, but none have yet been assessed in randomized, placebo-controlled designs. Ylvisaker, McPherson, Kayes, and Pellett (2008) developed a treatment they call "metaphoric identity mapping" and "identity-oriented goal setting (IOG)" aimed at integrating identity (and related motivational states) into goal setting and restructuring self-knowledge in a way that facilitates rehabilitation. Massimi et al. (2008) have used "in-home ambient computer display" to continuously play autobiographical information in the presence of a patient with AD. In a case study, they report that the treatment was associated with decreased apathy and more positive self-image.

One route to treatment of the self after brain injury might be to focus on social cognitive skills as these are skills that virtually all patients have difficulty with after brain injury.

Social-Cognitive Deficits in PD

Social cognition primarily involves attempts to model the beliefs, emotions, intentions, desires, and thoughts of other minds or persons (Anderson & Chen, 2002; Baldwin, 2003; Decety, 2007; Decety & Grèzes, 2006; Josephs & Ribbert, 2003; Keysers & Gazzola, 2007; Lieberman, 2007; Uddin, Iacoboni, & Lange, 2007). A key aspect of social cognition is, therefore, the ability to infer or simulate other people's mental states, thoughts, and feelings. This is sometimes referred to as theory of mind (ToM), or mentalizing ability. These mentalizing abilities both support and are supported by the so-called ECFs (Anderson & Chen, 2002; Baldwin, 2003; Decety, 2007; Decety & Grèzes, 2006; Josephs & Ribbert, 2003; Keysers & Gazzola, 2007; Lieberman, 2007; Uddin et al., 2007), such as attention, working memory, and planning processes. Both social cognitive and executive cognitive functions are impaired in PD (Crucian et al., 2001; Lange et al., 1993; Mathias, 2003; McNamara & Durso, 2003; McNamara, Durso, & Harris, 2006a,b, 2007; McNamara et al., 2003; Menza et al., 1993, 1995; Owen et al., 1992; Tomer & Aharon-Peretz, 2004).

Social Emotional Perception/Expression in PD

Communication of emotion between people is accomplished via several modalities including visual impressions, facial displays, speech, and gesture, to name a few. PD patients are impaired in many of these domains. Several recent studies (Kan, Kawamura, Hasegawa, Mochizuki, & Nakamura, 2002; Sprengelmeyer et al., 2003; Yip, Lee, Ho, Tsang, & Li, 2003) have reported that PD patients evidence impaired recognition of emotional expression in the faces of other people. This impairment persists even after controlling for visual discrimination deficits. Crucian et al. (2001) reported induction of verbal kinesia paradoxica in some patients with PD who were asked to recall emotional episodes. Patients could not adequately express their memory-linked emotions. All of these facts suggest that PD patients may be impaired in the expression and recognition of social emotions, and thus targeting social cognition in a rehabilitation program for PD will be a necessary component step in strengthening the agentic self in PD.

Social Cognition Interaction Training

A promising new rehabilitation program designed originally to help people with schizophrenia is called the Social Cognition Interaction Training (SCIT) program (Combs et al., 2007). SCIT is a manual-based, group intervention designed originally for individuals with schizophrenia spectrum disorders who evidenced deficits in the realm of social cognition. An examination of the exercises of the program suggests that it helps to strengthen the agentic self.

SCIT is a manual-based, 18-week group intervention composed of three phases: (1) understanding emotions (6 sessions); (2) social cognitive biases (7 sessions); and (3) integration (5 sessions). Group and homework exercises (spouses and caretakers are encouraged to assist in these homework exercises) promote social skill acquisition and maintenance over the 18-week intervention and beyond. One of the developers of SCIT, Dr. David Penn, professor of psychology at the University of North Carolina at Chapel Hill, in a private communication with me in 2007 said that SCIT can be and should be evaluated for clinical populations besides schizophrenics. PD patients, in particular, should be responsive to SCIT given the exercises it provides to strengthen agentic and executive aspects of the self.

The nonmotor social, cognitive, and neuropsychiatric disturbances associated with PD make SCIT a promising intervention for patients with PD who evidence neurocognitive and neuropsychiatric disturbances. In phase 1 of SCIT, we introduce social cognition by asking participants to discuss times when they have gotten social situations "wrong" (e.g., thinking someone was mad at them when they were not). The remainder of phase 1 is devoted to defining basic emotions and linking facial expressions to emotions. Phase 2 is devoted to strategies for avoiding the pitfalls associated with jumping to conclusions about people based on insufficient evidence. This concept is illustrated via videotaped interactions of actors who draw conclusions from events without having adequate information. One way to do this with PD patients is to tell them that one goal of the group program is to make them better social detectives, so as not to "convict" based on initial evidence, and so forth. To achieve this goal, patients are taught to brainstorm multiple possible explanations, first for positive events, and then for negative and ambiguous events. Events with ambiguous causes (e.g., you walk past a group of teenagers who start to laugh) are most problematic for patients with PD given their pragmatic and ToM deficits. So, special attention can be devoted to these sorts of exercises. Patients can be taught the differences between facts and guesses using photographs and videotapes. Emphasis can be placed on how guesses about social situations can impact feelings. Facts include objective situational variables (e.g., where people are located), statements made by people, facial expression or characteristics (e.g., color of hair), and so forth, whereas guesses are inferences about intangibles such as people's feelings, intentions, and motivations. This phase concludes with strategies to help participants make more conservative guesses and to better tolerate ambiguity. For example, participants may be asked to play "20 Questions" or to make bets about hypothetical social situations where uninformed guesses result in losing points. Putting these strategies in the context of games and betting is fun for participants and improves motivation. The final phase, Integration, is devoted to teaching participants to apply these social cognitive skills to their everyday lives. Participants practice using social cognitive strategies to interpret problematic situations that they have encountered and to plan appropriate steps to resolve them. Because this sort of intervention program has worked well with patients with schizophrenia, elements of it could be adopted to produce a program designed to strengthen the agentic self in PD via the targeting of social cognition. SCIT intensively challenges social skills and social cognitive skills of patients, and this likely has the effect of stimulating the agentic self as it is the self that acts in social situations. We have seen in the chapter on speech and language functions of PD (chapter 8) that PD patients evidence inordinate difficulty in comprehending speech-act verbs and phrases. Thus, a social cognitive rehabilitation program like SCIT will act to reinforce existing pragmatic language skills and to practice speech act comprehension skills that are weakening in PD.

The weakening of the agentic self in PD leads directly to all kinds of social interaction problems for patients with PD. Problematic social behaviors in PD patients have been documented repeatedly (Crucian et al., 2001; Mathias, 2003; Menza et al., 1993) and are a commonplace observation even in PD patients without frank neuropsychiatric disorders. In our clinical experience, for example, social deficits of PD involve social withdrawal, lack of interest and initiative in pursuing social interactions, inability to "read" emotional or facial expressions of others, personality and mood changes, occasional sexual improprieties, ignoring doctor's orders/suggestions, and a strange insensitivity to the social, moral, and personal consequences of inappropriate social behaviors. In addition, as reviewed throughout this book, nonmotor neuropsychiatric disturbances of PD include depression, anxiety, apathy, hallucinations, paranoid belief systems, and social withdrawal (Hubble & Koller, 1995; McNamara, Durso, Brown, & Lynch, 2003; Mendelsohn, Dakof, & Skaff, 1995; Saltzman et al., 2000). Certain social cognitive deficits of PD likely contribute to problematic social behaviors and neuropsychiatric disturbances of PD (Kaasinen et al., 2001; Lauterbach, 2005; Mathias, 2003; McNamara, Durso, & Harris, 2007). Thus, a rehabilitation program designed to improve both social cognition and the agentic self should be particularly helpful for these patients.

Cognitive Rehabilitation in PD

To my knowledge, only two studies have been published on attempts to implement a cognitive rehabilitation program for PD patients (Sammer, Reuter, Hullmann, Kaps, & Vaitl, 2006; Sinforiani, Banchieri, Zucchella, Pacchetti, & Sandrini, 2004). Sinforiani et al. (2004) assessed effects of a rehabilitation program of 6 weeks, including both motor and cognitive training, on 20 early-stage PD patients. The core of the program was repeated practice trials on computerized cognitive exercises. At the end of the 6-week training period, patients showed a significant improvement on verbal fluency, logical memory, and Raven's progressive matrices tests compared with baseline. Sammer et al. (2006) assessed effects of training on a range of executive function exercises over 10 treatment sessions (30 minutes each). The executive function treatment group demonstrated significant improvement relative to a control group on core executive abilities such as shifting set and organizing performance of a task even after controlling for depression, intelligence, and other potential confounders. Although the literature on cognitive rehabilitation in PD is scant, these two papers suggest that PD patients can benefit from standard techniques of cognitive rehabilitation.

It is very odd that so few cognitive rehabilitation interventions have been assessed in PD given the ubiquity of intervention programs that have been assessed in other clinical populations. Though none of these are aimed at strengthening the self, virtually all target ECFs in one way or another and thus should be valuable for PD. From the domain of TBI, three kinds of intervention have been assessed with randomized, placebo-controlled trial designs and found to be effective at improving ECFs in these populations. These are "training multiple steps," which included metacognitive strategy instruction (MSI); "training strategic thinking"; and "training multitasking." Notice that all three of these sorts of training programs are very clearly aimed at enhancing the ECF systems that normally support the agentic self. In MSI approaches, participants are trained to solve problems, to plan, or to be better organized by creating step-by-step procedures to accomplish a goal. To train to use strategic thinking, one also has to learn to multi-task and to self-regulate. Individuals need to identify an appropriate goal and predict their performance in advance of the activity, identify possible solutions based on past experience, monitor progress toward the goal, and adjust performance when necessary. These are the functions of the agentic self that I noted in previous chapters: identifying values, choosing values to be pursued, making predictions about potential success, self-monitoring performance during activities, using mental simulation capacities to evaluate the usefulness of solutions and strategies and to generate alternative solutions, then developing plans to attain a goal, and so forth.

Summary

The review of the literature and our own clinical experience suggests that one of the most severe and disabling cognitive sequelae of PD lies in the realm of the agentic self and *social cognition*—yet no well-studied program of rehabilitation of these deficits yet exists for PD patients. Developing effective rehabilitation programs for social cognitive and executive functions of PD is of fundamental clinical and theoretical importance because neuropsychiatric dysfunction in PD increases caregiver burden, reduces quality of life, and may compromise complex decision-making capacities around long-term care. Changes in interpersonal, personality, and social functions, furthermore, may predate onset of overt extrapyramidal motor signs of PD by several years, and thus targeting these deficits for retraining may help in maintaining independence over a longer period of time.

PD has to be understood as a disorder of the whole person. It is a disorder of action, and only a person can act. There is an emerging consensus within neuropsychology that to really harness an individual's coping powers, one has to address the person—the self—who is in crisis due to illness or injury. Several developments within the neurosciences have forced clinicians and scientists to finally take the person, the self, seriously. The development of the field of social neuroscience has shown us how the self and its capacities can be rigorously measured without having to have a complete theory of the self. Functional neuroimaging techniques and related cognitive neuroscience methods have demonstrated that a minimal self and an agentic self can be characterized and associated with consistent sets of neural networks. Advances in the psychological sciences have demonstrated that behaviors, emotions, and mental content cannot be fully understood without reference to a self, or at least a small set of selves, who experience the emotions or mental content and who use the information to implement strategically informed decisions and actions. Developments within the human sciences, more generally, have emphasized the capacities of human persons to actively construct meaning in the context of interactions with others. Meaning only makes sense in relation to events that happen to individual persons who interact with other persons. In short, there is now a broad consensus developing within the human sciences and neurosciences that selves are necessary entities or constructs that we must assume exist to understand human behavior and actions. They are particularly important for theories of how people survive and cope with disease, including Parkinson's disease.

References

Aarsland, D., & Kurz, M. W. (2010). The epidemiology of dementia associated with Parkinson disease. *Journal of the Neurological Sciences, 289*(1–2), 18–22.

Aarsland, D., Larsen, J. P., Lim, N. G., Janvin, C., Karlsen, K., Tandberg, E., et al. (1999). Range of neuropsychiatric disturbances in patients with Parkinson's disease. *Journal of Neurology, Neurosurgery, and Psychiatry, 67*, 492–496.

Aarsland, D., Litvan, I., Galasko, D., Wentzel-Larsen, T., & Larsen, J. P. (2003). Performance on the dementia rating scale in Parkinson's disease with dementia and dementia with Lewy bodies: Comparison with progressive supranuclear palsy and Alzheimer's disease. *Journal of Neurology, Neurosurgery, and Psychiatry, 74*, 1215–1220.

Abbott, R. D., Ross, G. W., Petrovitch, H., Tanner, C. M., Davis, D. G., Masaki, K. H., et al. (2007). Bowel movement frequency in late-life and incidental Lewy bodies. *Movement Disorders, 22*(11), 1581–1586.

Abe, N., Fujii, T., Hirayama, K., Takeda, A., Hosokai, Y., Ishioka, T., et al. (2009). Do parkinsonian patients have trouble telling lies? The neurobiological basis of deceptive behavior. *Brain, 132*(5), 1386–1395.

Adolphs, R., Tranel, D., Damasio, H., & Damasio, A. (1994). Impaired recognition of emotion in facial expressions following bilateral damage to the human amygdala. *Nature, 372*, 669–672.

Agargun, M. Y., Cilli, A. S., Kara, H., Tarhan, N., Kincir, F., & Oz, H. (1998). Repetitive frightening dreams and suicidal behavior in patients with major depression. *Comprehensive Psychiatry, 39*, 198–202.

Agargun, M. Y., Kara, H., & Solmaz, M. (2007). Sleep disturbance and suicidal behavior in patients with major depression. *Journal of Clinical Psychiatry, 58*(6), 249–251.

Aggleton, J. P. (2000). *The amygdala: A functional analysis.* Oxford, UK: Oxford University Press.

Agid, Y., Javoy-Agid, M., & Ruberg, M. (1987). Biochemistry of neurotransmitters in Parkinson's disease. In C. D. Marsden & S. Fahn (Eds.), *Movement disorders 2* (pp. 166–230). New York: Butterworth & Co.

Ahearn, L. M. (2001). Language and agency. *Annual Review of Anthropology, 30*, 109–137.

Aldrich, M. S. (2000). Parkinsonism. In M. H. Kryger, T. Roth, & W. C. Dement (Eds.), *Principles and practice of sleep medicine* (3rd ed., pp. 1051–1057). Philadelphia: W. B. Saunders.

Alfimova, M., Golimbet, V., Gritsenk, I., Lezheiko, T., Abramova, L., Strel'tsova, M., et al. (2007). Interaction of dopamine system genes and cognitive functions in patients with schizophrenia and their relatives and in healthy subjects from the general population. *Neuroscience and Behavioral Physiology, 37*, 643–651.

Altgassen, M., Zöllig, J., Kopp, U., Mackinlay, R., & Kliegel, M. (2007). Patients with Parkinson's disease can successfully remember to execute delayed intentions. *Journal of the International Neuropsychological Society, 13*, 888–892.

American Psychiatric Association. (2000). *Diagnostic and statistical manual of mental disorders* (4th ed., text rev.). Washington, DC: Author.

Amick, M. M., Grace, J., & Chou, K. L. (2006). Body side of motor symptom onset in Parkinson's disease is associated with memory performance. *Journal of Neurology, Neurosurgery, and Psychiatry, 12,* 736–740.

Amin, F., Davidson, M., & Davis, K. L. (1992). Homovanillic acid measurement in clinical research: A review of methodology. *Schizophrenia Bulletin, 18*(1), 123–148.

Anderson, S. M., & Chen, S. (2002). The relational self: An interpersonal social-cognitive theory. *Psychological Review, 109*(4), 619–645.

Angwin, A. J., Chenery, H. J., Copland, D. A., Murdoch, B. E., & Silburn, P. A. (2006). Self-paced reading and sentence comprehension in Parkinson's disease. *Journal of Neurolinguistics, 19*(3), 239–252.

Armitage, R. (2007). Sleep and circadian rhythms in mood disorders. *Acta Psychiatrica Scandinavica, 115*(S433), 104–115.

Arnott, W. L., Chenery, H. J., Murdoch, B. E., & Silburn, P. A. (2005). Morphosyntactic and syntactic priming: An investigation of underlying processing mechanisms and the effects of Parkinson's disease. *Journal of Neurolinguistics, 18*(1), 1–28.

Arnulf, I., Bonnet, A. M., Damier, P., Bejjani, B. P., Seilhean, D., Derenne, J. P., et al. (2000). Hallucinations, REM sleep, and Parkinson's disease: A medical hypothesis. *Neurology, 55*(2), 281–288.

Austin, J. L. (1962). *How to do things with words.* Oxford, UK: Clarendon Press.

Badre, D. (2008). Cognitive control, hierarchy, and the rostro-caudal organization of the frontal lobes. *Trends in Cognitive Sciences, 12*(5), 193–200.

Badre, D., & D'Esposito, M. (2007). Functional magnetic resonance imaging evidence for a hierarchical organization of the prefrontal cortex. *Journal of Cognitive Neuroscience, 199,* 2082–2099.

Baldwin, M. W. (2003). *Interpersonal cognition.* New York: The Guilford Press.

Bandura, A. (1989). Human agency in social cognitive theory. *American Psychologist, 44,* 1175–1184.

Banyas, C. A. (1999). Evolution and phylogenetic history of the frontal lobes. In B. L. Miller & J. L. Cummings (Eds.), *The human frontal lobes: Functions and disorders* (pp. 83–106). New York: The Guilford Press.

Bara, B. G., Tirassa, M., & Zettin, M. (1997). Neuropragmatics: neuropsychological constraints on formal theories of dialogue. *Brain and Language, 59,* 7–49.

Barton, R. A., & Harvey, P. H. (2000). Mosaic evolution of brain structure in mammals. *Nature, 405,* 1055–1058.

Baumeister, R., & Vohs, K. (Eds.). (2004). *Handbook of self-regulation: Research, theory and applications.* New York: The Guilford Press.

Baxter, L. R., Schwartz, J. M., Phelps, M. E., Mazziotta, J. C., Guze, B. H., Selin, C. E., et al. (1989). Reduction of prefrontal cortex glucose metabolism common to three types of depression. *Archives of General Psychiatry, 46,* 243–250.

Bayles, K. A., Tomoeda, C. K., Wood, J. A., Montgomery, E. B., Jr., Cruz, R. F., Azuma, T., et al. (1996). Change in cognitive function in idiopathic Parkinson disease. *Archives of Neurology, 53*(11), 1140–1146.

Bechara, A., Damasio, A. R., Damasio, H., & Anderson, S. W. (1994). Insensitivity to future consequences following damage to human prefrontal cortex. *Cognition, 50,* 7–15.

Bechara, A., Damasio, H., Tranel, D., & Damasio, A. R. (1997). Deciding advantageously before knowing the advantageous strategy. *Science, 275,* 1293–1295.

Bedard, M. A., el Massioui, F., Malapani, C., Dubois, B., Pillon, B., Renault, B., et al. (1998). Attentional deficits in Parkinson's disease: Partial reversibility with naphtoxazine (SDZ NVI-085), a selective noradrenergic alpha 1 agonist. *Clinical Neuropharmacology, 21,* 108–117.

Belicki, K. (1986). Recalling dreams: An examination of daily variation and individual differences. In J. Gackenbach (Ed.), *Sleep and dreams: A sourcebook* (pp. 187–206). New York: Garland.

Bell, D. E. (1982). Regret in decision making under uncertainty. *Operations Research, 30*, 961–981.

Benca, R. M. (2000). Mood disorders. In M. H. Kryger, T. Roth, & W. C. Dement (Eds.), *Principles and practice of sleep medicine* (3rd ed., pp. 1140–1148). Philadelphia: W. B. Saunders.

Ben-Yishay, Y., Rattok, J., Lakin, P., Piasetsky, E. D., Ross, B., Silver, S., et al. (1985). Neuropsychologic rehabilitation: Quest for a holistic approach. *Seminars in Neurology, 5*, 252–259.

Benjamin, R., & Golden, G. T. (1985). Extent and organization of opossum prefrontal cortex defined by anterograde and retrograde transport methods. *Journal of Comparative Neurology, 238*, 77–91.

Biary, N., & Koller, W. (1985). Handedness and essential tremor. *Archives of Neurology, 42*(11), 1082–1083.

Blakemore, S. J., Frith, C. D., & Wolpert, D. M. (2001). The cerebellum is involved in predicting the sensory consequences of action. *Neuroreport, 12*(9), 1879–1884.

Blakemore, S-J., Smith, J., Steel, R., Johnstone, E., & Frith, C. D. (2000). The perception of self-produced sensory stimuli in patients with auditory hallucinations and passivity experiences: Evidence for a breakdown in self-monitoring. *Psychological Medicine, 30*, 1131–1139.

Blinkov, S. M., & Glezer, I. I. (1968). *The human brain in figures and tables*. New York: Plenum Press.

Bliwise, D. L. (2000). Normal aging. In M. H. Kryger, T. Roth, & W. C. Dement (Eds.), *Principles and practice of sleep medicine* (3rd ed., pp. 26–42). Philadelphia: W. B. Saunders.

Bodden, M. E., Mollenhauer, B., Trenkwalder, C., Cabanel, N., Eggert, K. M., Unger, M. M., et al. (2010). Affective and cognitive theory of mind in patients with Parkinson's disease. *Parkinsonism & Related Disorders, 16*(7), 466–470.

Boeve, B. F., Silber, M. H., Ferman, T. J., Lucas, J. A., & Parisi, J. E. (2001). Association of REM sleep behavior disorder and neurodegenerative disease may reflect an underlying synucleinopathy. *Movement Disorders, 16*(4), 622–630.

Bohnen, N. I., Kaufer, D. I., Ivanco, L. S., Lopresti, B., Koeppe, R. A., Davis, J. G., et al. (2003). Cortical cholinergic function is more severely affected in parkinsonian dementia than in Alzheimer disease: An in vivo positron emission tomographic study. *Archives of Neurology, 60*, 1745–1748.

Bonnet, M. H. (2000). Sleep deprivation. In M. H. Kryger, T. Roth, & W. C. Dement (Eds.), *Principles and practice of sleep medicine* (3rd ed., pp. 53–71). Philadelphia: W. B. Saunders.

Booth, G. (1948). Psychodynamics in Parkinsonism. *Psychosomatic Medicine, 10*, 1–14.

Borbely, A. (1984). Schlafgewohnheiten, Schlafqualität und Schlafmittelkonsum der Schweizer Bevölkerung: Ergebnisse einer Repräsentativumfrage. *Schweizerische Arztezeitung, 65*, 1606–1613.

Borckardt, J. J., Smith, A. R., Reeves, S. T., Weinstein, M., Kozel, F. A., Nahas, Z., et al. (2007). Fifteen minutes of left prefrontal repetitive transcranial magnetic stimulation acutely increases thermal pain thresholds in healthy *adults*. *Pain Research & Management, 12*, 287–290.

Botvinick, M. M. (2008). Hierarchical models of behavior and prefrontal function. *Trends in Cognitive Sciences, 12*, 201–208.

Boulenger, V., Mechtouff, L., Thobois, S., Broussolle, E., Jeannerod, M., & Nazir, T. A. (2008). Word processing in Parkinson's disease is impaired for action verbs but not for concrete nouns. *Neuropsychologia, 46*(2), 743–756.

Bower, J. H., Grossardt, B. R., Maraganore, D. M., Ahlskog, J. E., Colligan, R. C., Geda, Y. E., et al. (2010). Anxious personality predicts an increased risk of Parkinson's disease. *Movement Disorders, 25*(13), 2105–2113.

Boyer, P., Robbins, P., & Jack, A. (2005). Varieties of self-systems worth having. *Consciousness and Cognition, 14*, 647–660.

Braak, H., Ghebremedhin, E., Rüb, U., Bratzke, H., & Del Tredici, K. (2004). Stages in the development of Parkinson's disease-related pathology. *Cell and Tissue Research, 318*(1), 121–134.

Brand, M., Labudda, K., Kalbe, E., Hilker, R., Emmans, D., Fuchs, G., et al. (2004). Decision-making impairments in patients with Parkinson's disease. *Behavioural Neurology, 15*, 77–85.

Braun, A. R., Balkin, T. J., Wesenstein, N. J., Varga, M., Baldwin, P., Selbie, S., et al. (1997). Regional cerebral blood flow throughout the sleep-wake cycle. *Brain, 120*, 1173–1197.

Braun, M., & Muermann, A. (2004). .The impact of regret on the demand for insurance. *Journal of Risk and Insurance, 71*(4), 737–767.

Brody, A. L., Saxena, S., Silverman, D. H. S., Alborzian, S., Fairbanks, L. A., Maidment, K. M., et al. (1999). Brain metabolic changes in major depressive disorder from pre- to post-treatment with paroxetine. *Psychiatry Research: Neuroimaging, 91*, 127–139.

Brønnick, K., Emre, M., Lane, R., Tekin, S., & Aarsland, D. (2007). Profile of cognitive impairment in dementia associated with Parkinson's disease compared with Alzheimer's disease. *Journal of Neurology, Neurosurgery, and Psychiatry, 78*, 1064–1068.

Brooks, D. N., & McKinlay, W. (1983). Personality and behavioral changes after severe blunt head injury: A relative's view. *Journal of Neurology, Neurosurgery, and Psychiatry, 46*, 333–334.

Brown, P., & Levinson, S. (1987). *Politeness: Some universals in language usage.* Cambridge, UK: Cambridge University Press.

Brozoski, T. J., Brown, R. M., Rosvold, H. E., & Goldman, P. S. (1979). Cognitive deficit caused by regional depletion of dopamine in prefrontal cortex of rhesus monkey. *Science, 205*, 929–932.

Bruner, J. (1995). The autobiographical process. *Current Sociology, 43*, 161–177.

Bunney, B. S., Chiodo, L. A., & Grace, A. A. (1991). Midbrain dopamine system electrophysiological functioning: A review and new hypothesis. *Synapse (New York, N.Y.), 9*(2), 79–94.

Burgess, P. W., Gilbert, S. J., & Dumontheil, I. (2007). Function and localization within rostral prefrontal cortex (area 10). *Philosophical Transactions of the Royal Society, B, 362*, 887–899.

Burgess, P. W., Scott, S. K., & Frith, C. D. (2003). The role of the rostral frontal cortex (in area 10) in prospective memory: A lateral versus medial dissociation. *Neuropsychologia, 41*, 906–918.

Burns, K., & Bechara, A. (2007). Decision making and free will: A neuroscience perspective. *Behavioral Sciences & the Law, 25*(2), 263–280.

Burton, E. J., McKeith, I. G., Burn, D. J., Williams, E. D., & O'Brien, J. T. (2004). Cerebral atrophy in Parkinson's disease with and without dementia: A comparison with Alzheimer's disease, dementia with Lewy bodies and controls. *Brain, 127*(Pt 4), 791–800.

Bush, E. C., & Allman, J. M. (2004). The scaling of frontal cortex in primates and carnivores. *Proceedings of the National Academy of Sciences of the United States of America, 101*, 3962–3966.

Butler, P. M., & McNamara, P. (2011). Epigenetic, imprinting and neurobehavioral effects in Parkinson's disease. In P. McNamara (Ed.), *Dementia: Volume 2: Science and biology.* Santa Barbara, CA: Praeger Publishers. In press.

Buzsáki, G. (1996). The hippocampo-neocortical dialogue. *Cerebral Cortex, 6*, 81–92.

Byrne, R. M. J. (1997). Cognitive processes in counterfactual thinking about what might have been. *The Psychology of Learning and Motivation, 37*, 105–154.

Caap-Ahlgren, M., & Dehlin, O. (2002). Factors of importance to the caregiver burden experienced by family caregivers of Parkinson's disease patients. *Aging Clinical and Experimental Research, 14*(5), 371–377.

Camperio Ciani, A. S., Capiluppi, C., Veronese, A., & Sartori, G. (2007). The adaptive value of personality differences revealed by small island population dynamics. *European Journal of Personality, 21*, 3–22.

Canli, T. (2006). *Biology of personality and individual differences.* New York: The Guilford Press.

Caparros-Lefebvre, D., Pecheux, N., Petit, V., Duhamel, A., & Petit, H. (1995). Which factors predict cognitive decline in Parkinson's disease? *Journal of Neurology, Neurosurgery, and Psychiatry*, *58*(1), 51–55.

Carskadon, M. A., & Dement, W. C. (2000). Normal human sleep: An overview. In M. H. Kryger, T. Roth, & W. C. Dement (Eds.), *Principles and practice of sleep medicine* (3rd ed., pp. 15–25). Philadelphia: W. B. Saunders.

Chang, F. M., Kidd, J. R., Livak, K. J., Pakstis, A. J., & Kidd, K. K. (1996). The worldwide distribution of allele frequencies at the human dopamine D4 receptor locus. *Human Genetics*, *98*, 91–101.

Chen, C., Burton, M. L., Greenberger, E., & Dmitrieva, J. (1999). Population migration and the variation of dopamine D4 receptor (DRD4) allele frequencies around the Globe. *Evolution and Human Behavior*, *20*, 309–324.

Christie, R., & Geis, F. L. (Eds.). (1970). *Studies in Machiavellianism*. New York: Academic Press.

Christoff, K., & Gabrieli, J. D. E. (2000). The frontopolar cortex and human cognition: Evidence for a rostrocaudal hierarchical organization within the human prefrontal cortex. *Psychobiology*, *28*, 168–186.

Churchland, P. S. (2002). Self-representation in the nervous system. *Science*, *296*, 308–310.

Clark, H. H. (1996). *Using language*. Cambridge, UK: Cambridge University Press.

Cloute, K., Mitchell, A., & Yates, P. (2008). Traumatic brain injury and the construction of identity: A discursive approach. *Neuropsychological Rehabilitation*, *18*(5–6), 651–670.

Cohen, A. L., & Gollwitzer, P. M. (2007). The cost of remembering to remember: Cognitive load and implementation intentions influence ongoing task performance. In M. Kliegel, M. McDaniel, & G. Einstein (Eds.), *Prospective memory: Cognitive, neuroscience, developmental, and applied perspectives* (pp. 367–390). Mahwah, NJ: Erlbaum.

Cohen, P. R., Morgan, J., & Pollack, M. E. (Eds.). (1990). *Intentions in communication*. Cambridge, MA: The MIT Press.

Colman, K., Koerts, J., van Beilen, M., Leenders, K. L., & Bastiaanse, R. (2006). The role of cognitive mechanisms in sentence comprehension in Dutch speaking Parkinson's disease patients: Preliminary data. *Brain and Language*, *99*, 120–121.

Combs, D. R., Adams, S. D., Penn, D. L., Roberts, D., Tiegreen, J., & Stem, P. (2007). Social Cognition and Interaction Training (SCIT) for inpatients with schizophrenia spectrum disorders: Preliminary findings. *Schizophrenia Research*, *91*(1–3), 112–116.

Comings, D. E., Gonzalez, N., Wu, S., Gade, R., Muhleman, D., Saucier, G., et al. (1999). Studies of the 48 bp repeat polymorphism of the DRD4 gene in impulsive, compulsive, addictive behaviors: Tourette syndrome, ADHD, pathological gambling, and substance abuse. *American Journal of Medical Genetics*, *88*(4), 358–368.

Comrie, B. (1981). *Language universals and linguistic typology: Syntax and morphology*. Oxford, UK: Blackwell.

Cools, R., Stefanova, E., Barker, R. A., Robins, T. W., & Owen, A. M. (2002). Dopaminergic modulation of high level cognition in Parkinson's disease: The role of the prefrontal cortex revealed by PET. *Brain*, *125*, 584–594.

Cooper-Evans, S., Alderman, N., Knight, C., & Oddy, M. (2008). Self-esteem as a predictor of psychological distress after severe acquired brain injury: An exploratory study. *Neuropsychological Rehabilitation*, *18*(5–6), 607–626.

Corballis, M. C. (2002). *From hand to mouth: the origins of language*. Princeton, NJ: Princeton University Press.

Costello, S., Cockburn, N., Bronstein, J., Zhang, X., & Ritz, B. (2009). Parkinson's disease and residential exposure to maneb and paraquat from agricultural applications in the Central Valley of California. *American Journal of Epidemiology*, *169*(8), 919–926.

Cotelli, M., Borroni, B., Manenti, R., Zanetti, M., Arevalo, A., Cappa, S. F., et al. (2007). Action and object naming in Parkinson's disease without dementia. *European Journal of Neurology, 14,* 632–637.

Crucian, G. P., Huang, L., Barrett, A. M., Schwartz, R. L., Cibula, J. E., Anderson, J. M., et al. (2001). Emotional conversations in Parkinson's disease. *Neurology, 56,* 159–165.

Culbertson, W. C., Moberg, P. J., Duda, J. E., Stern, M. B., & Weintraub, D. (2004). Assessing the executive function deficits of patients with Parkinson's disease: Utility of the Tower of London-Drexel. *Assessment, 11*(1), 27–39.

Cummings, J. L. (1992). Depression and Parkinson's disease: A review. *American Journal of Psychiatry, 149*(4), 443–454.

Cummings, J. L. (1997). The Neuropsychiatric Inventory: Assessing psychopathology in dementia patients. *Neurology, 48*(Suppl. 6), S10–S16.

Czernecki, V., Pillon, B., Houeto, J. L., Pochon, B., Levy, R., & Dubois, R. (2002). Motivation, reward, and Parkinson's disease: Influence of dopatherapy. *Neuropsychologia, 40,* 2257–2267.

DATATOP Study. (1996). Impact of deprenyl and tocopherol treatment on Parkinson's disease in DATATOP subjects not requiring levodopa. Parkinson Study Group. *Annals of Neurology, 39*(1), 29–36.

Davidson, R. J. (2002). Anxiety and affective style: Role of prefrontal cortex and amygdala. *Biological Psychiatry, 51,* 29–37.

Deacon, T. W. (1990). Fallacies of progression in theories of brain-size evolution. *International Journal of Primatology, 11,* 193–236.

Decety, J. (2007). A social cognitive neuroscience model of human empathy. In E. Harmon-Jones & P. Winkielman (Eds.), *Social neuroscience: Integrating biological and psychological explanations of social behavior* (pp. 246–270). New York: The Guilford Press.

Decety, J., & Grèzes, J. (2006). The power of simulation: Imagining one's own and other's behavior. *Brain Research, 1079*(1), 4–14.

Delazer, M., Sinz, H., Zamarian, L., Stockner, H., Seppi, K., Wenning, G. K., et al. (2009). Decision making under risk and under ambiguity in Parkinson's disease. *Neuropsychologia, 47,* 1901–1908.

Delis, D. C., Kaplan, E., & Kramer, J. H. (2001). *Delis Kaplan executive function system: Technical manual.* San Antonio, TX: Psychological Corporation.

Demet, E. M., Chicz-Demet, A., Fallon, J. H., & Sokolski, K. N. (1999). Sleep deprivation therapy in depressive illness and Parkinson's disease. *Progress in Neuro-Psychopharmacology & Biological Psychiatry, 23,* 753–784.

Depue, R. A. (2006). Interpersonal behavior and the structure of personality: Neurobehavioral foundation of agentic extraversion and affiliation. In T. Canli (Ed.), *Biology of personality and individual differences* (pp. 60–92). New York: The Guilford Press.

Dethy, S., Van Blercom, N., Damhaut, P., Wilder, D., Hildebrand, J., & Goldman, S. (1998). Asymmetry of basal ganglia glucose metabolism and dopa responsiveness in parkinsonism. *Movement Disorders, 13,* 275–280.

Dinges, D. F., Pack, F., Williams, K., Gillen, K. A., Powell, J. W., Ott, G. E., et al. (1997). Cumulative sleepiness, mood disturbance, and psychomotor vigilance performance decrements during a week of sleep restricted to 4–5 hours per night. *Sleep, 20*(4), 267–277.

Direnfeld, L. K., Albert, M. L., Volicer, L., Langlais, P. J., Marquis, J., & Kaplan, E. (1984). Parkinson's disease. The possible relationship of laterality to dementia and neurochemical findings. *Archives of Neurology, 41*(9), 935–941.

Divac, I., Holst, M. C., Nelson, J., & McKenzie, J. S. (1987). Afferents of the frontal cortex in the echidna (*Tachyglossus aculeatus*): Indication of an outstandingly large prefrontal area. *Brain, Behavior and Evolution, 30,* 303–320.

Divac, I., Pettigrew, J. D., Holst, M.-C., & McKenzie, J. S. (1987). Efferent connections of the prefrontal cortex of echidna. *Brain, Behavior and Evolution, 30,* 321–327.

Dixon, R. M. W. (1994). *Ergativity.* New York: Cambridge University Press.

Djaldetti, R., Shifrin, A., Rogowski, Z., Sprecher, E., Melamed, E., & Yarnitsky, D. (2004). Quantitative measurement of pain sensation in patients with Parkinson disease. *Neurology, 62,* 2171–2217.

Djaldetti, R., Ziv, I., & Melamed, E. (2006). The mystery of motor asymmetry in Parkinson's disease. *Lancet Neurology, 5*(9), 796–802.

Domhoff, G. W. (1996). *Finding meaning in dreams: A quantitative approach.* New York: Plenum Press.

Downes, J. J., Sharp, H. M., Costall, B. M., Sagar, H. J., & Howe, J. (1993). Alternating fluency in Parkinson's disease. *Brain, 116,* 887–902.

Drake, D. F., Harkins, S., & Qutubuddin, A. (2005). Pain in Parkinson's disease: Pathology to treatment, medication to deep brain stimulation. *NeuroRehabilitation, 20*(4), 335–341.

Drevets, W. C. (2007). Orbitofrontal cortex function and structure in depression. *Annals of the New York Academy of Sciences, 1121,* 499–527.

Drevets, W. C., & Price, J. L. (2005). Neuroimaging and neuropathological studies of mood disorders. In J. W. M. Licinio (Ed.), *Biology of depression: From novel insights to therapeutic strategies* (pp. 427–466). Weinheim, Germany: Wiley-VCH.

Drevets, W. C., Price, J. L., Bardgett, M. E., Reich, T., Todd, R. D., & Raichle, M. E. (2002). Glucose metabolism in the amygdala in depression: Relationship to diagnostic subtype and plasma cortisol levels. *Pharmacology Biology and Behavior, 71,* 431–447.

Drevets, W. C., Price, J. L., Simpson, J. R., Jr., Todd, R. D., Reich, T., Vannier, M., et al. (1997). Subgenual prefrontal cortex abnormalities in mood disorders. *Nature, 386,* 824–827.

Drevets, W. C., Videen, T. O., Price, J. L., Preskorn, S. H., Carmichael, S. T., & Raichle, M. E. (1992). A functional anatomical study of unipolar depression. *Journal of Neuroscience, 12,* 3628–3641.

D'Souza, U. M., Russ, C., Tahir, E., Mill, J., McGuffin, P., Asherson, P., et al. (2004). Functional effects of a tandem duplication polymorphism in the 5 prime flanking region of the DRD4 gene. *Biological Psychiatry, 56,* 691–697.

Dubois, B., Boller, F., Pillon, B., & Agid, Y. (1991). Cognitive deficits in Parkinson's disease. In F. Boller & J. Grafman (Eds.), *Handbook of neuropsychology* (Vol. 5, pp. 195–240). Amsterdam, The Netherlands: Elsevier.

Dujardin, K., Sockeel, P., Delliaux, M., Destée, A., & Defebvre, L. (2009). Apathy may herald cognitive decline and dementia in Parkinson's disease. *Movement Disorders, 24*(16), 2391–2397.

Dujardin, K., Sockeel, P., Devos, D., Delliaux, M., Krystkowiak, P., Destée, A., et al. (2007). Characteristics of apathy in Parkinson's disease. *Movement Disorders, 22*(6), 778–784.

Dulawa, S. C., Grandy, D. K., Low, M. J., Paulus, M. P., & Geyer, M. A. (1999). Dopamine D4 receptor-knock-out mice exhibit reduced exploration of novel stimuli. *Journal of Neuroscience, 19,* 9550–9556.

Durstewitz, D., & Seamans, J. K. (2008). The dual-state theory of prefrontal cortex dopamine function with relevance to catechol-o-methyltransferase genotypes and schizophrenia. *Biological Psychiatry, 64*(9), 739–749.

Duvoisin, R. C., Eldridge, R., Williams, A., Nutt, J., & Calne, O. (1981). Twin study of Parkinson disease. *Neurology, 31*(1), 77.

Eatough, V. M., Kempster, P. A., Stern, G. M., & Lees, A. J. (1990). Premorbid personality and idiopathic Parkinson's disease. *Advances in Neurology, 53,* 335–337.

Ebert, D., Feistel, H., & Barocka, A. (1991). Effects of sleep deprivation on the limbic system and the frontal lobes in affective disorders: A study with Tc-99m-HMPAO SPECT. *Psychiatry Reasearch: NeuroImaging, 40,* 247–251.

Ebert, D., Feistel, H., Barocka, A., & Kaschka, W. (1994). Increased limbic blood flow and total sleep deprivation in major depression with melancholia. *Psychiatry Research: Neuroimaging, 55,* 101–109.

Ebert, D., Feistel, H., Kaschka, W., Barocka, A., & Pirner, A. (1994). Single photon emission computerized tomography assessment of cerebral dopamine D2 receptor blockade in depression before and after sleep deprivation—Preliminary results. *Biological Psychiatry, 35,* 880–885.

Ebstein, R. P. (2006). The molecular genetic architecture of human personality: Beyond self-report questionnaires. *Molecular Psychiatry, 11,* 427–445.

Edwards, N. E., & Scheetz, P. S. (2002). Predictors of burden for caregivers of patients with Parkinson's disease. *Journal of Neuroscience Nursing, 34*(4), 184–190.

Einstein, G. O., McDaniel, M. A., Thomas, R., Mayfield, S., Shank, H., Morisette, N., et al. (2005). Multiple processes in prospective memory retrieval: Factors determining monitoring versus spontaneous retrieval. *Journal of Experimental Psychology: General, 134,* 327–342.

Elbaz, A., Bower, J. H., Peterson, B. J., Maraganore, D. M., McDonnell, S. K., Ahlskog, E., et al. (2003). Survival study of Parkinson disease in Olmsted County, Minnesota. *Archives of Neurology, 60,* 91–96.

Elsworth, J. D., Leahy, D. J., Roth, R. H., & Redmond, D. E., Jr. (1987). Homovanillic acid concentrations in brain, CSF and plasma as indicators of central dopamine function in primates. *Journal of Neural Transmission, 68,* 51–62.

Emre, M. (2003). What causes mental dysfunction in Parkinson's disease? *Movement Disorders, 18* (Suppl. 6), 563–571.

Emre, M., Aarsland, D., Albanese, A., Byrne, E. J., Deuschl, G., De Deyn, P. P., et al. (2004). Rivastigmine for dementia associated with Parkinson's disease. *New England Journal of Medicine, 351*(24), 2509–2518.

Emre, M., Aarsland, D., Brown, R., Burn, D. J., Duyckaerts, C., Mizuno, Y., et al. (2007). Clinical diagnostic criteria for dementia associated with Parkinson's disease. *Movement Disorders, 22,* 1689–1707.

Euteneuer, F., Boucsein, W., Schaefer, F., Stürmer, R., Timmermann, L., Barbe, M., et al. (2009). Dissociation of decision-making under ambiguity and decision-making under risk in patients with Parkinson's disease: A neuropsychological and psychophysiological study. *Neuropsychologia, 47,* 2882–2890.

Fahn, S. Elton, R. L., and members of the UPDRS Development Committee. (1987). Unified Parkinson's Disease Rating Scale. In S. Fahn, C. D. Marsden, M. Goldstein, & D. B. Calne (Eds.), *Recent developments in Parkinson's disease* (pp. 153–163). New York: Macmillan.

Fantini, M. L., Corona, A., Clerici, S., & Ferini-Strambi, L. (2005). Aggressive dream content without daytime aggressiveness in REM sleep behavior disorder. *Neurology, 65*(7), 1010–1015.

Farrar, C., & Frith, C. D. (2002). Experiencing oneself vs another person as being the cause of an action: The neural correlates of the experience of agency. *NeuroImage, 15*(3), 596–603.

Farrer, C., Franck, N., Georgieff, N., Frith, C. D., Decety, J., & Jeannerod, M. (2003). Modulating the experience of agency: A positron emission tomography study. *NeuroImage, 18*(2), 324–333.

Feinberg, T., & Keenan, J. (Eds.). (2005). *The lost self: Pathologies of the brain and identity.* Oxford, UK: Oxford University Press.

Fernandez, H., & Durso, R. (1998). Clozapine for the treatment of dopaminergic-induced paraphilias in Parkinson disease. *Movement Disorders, 13*(3), 597–598.

Fink, G. R., Marshall, J. C., Halligan, P. W., Frith, C. D., Driver, J., Frackowiak, R. S., et al. (1999). The neural consequences of conflict between intention and the sense. *Brain, 122*(Pt 3), 497–512.

Finlay, B. L., & Darlington, R. B. (1995). Linked regularities in the development and evolution of mammalian brains. *Science, 268*(5217), 1578–1584.

Finlay, B. L., Darlington, R. B., & Nicastro, N. (2001). Developmental structure in brain evolution. *Behavioral and Brain Sciences, 24*(2), 263–278.

Foley, W. A. (1999). Information structure. In K. Brown, & J. Miller (Eds.) & R. E. Asher (Consulting Ed.), *Concise encyclopedia of grammatical categories* (pp. 204–213). Amsterdam, The Netherlands: Elsevier.

Folstein, M., Folstein, S., & McHugh, P. (1975). "Mini-mental state": A practical method for grading the cognitive state of patients for the clinician. *Journal of Psychiatric Research, 12*, 189–198.

Fotopoulou, A. (2008). False-selves in neuropsychological rehabilitation: The challenge of confabulation. *Neuropsychological Rehabilitation, 18*(5–6), 541–565.

Friederici, A. D., Kotz, S. A., Werheid, K., Hein, G., & von Cramon, D. Y. (2003). Syntactic comprehension in Parkinson's disease: Investigating early automatic and late integrational processes using event-related brain potentials. *Neuropsychology, 17*, 133–142.

Frith, C. D. (2005). The self in action: Lessons from delusions of control. *Consciousness and Cognition, 14*, 752–770.

Froehlicha, T. E., Lanpheara, B. P., Dietrichb, K. N., Cory-Slechtac, D. A., Wanga, N., & Kahna, R. S. (2007). Interactive effects of a DRD4 polymorphism, lead, and sex on executive functions in children. *Biological Psychiatry, 62*(3), 234–249.

Frucht, S., Rogers, J. D., Greene, P. E., Gordon, M. F., & Fahn, S. (1999). Falling asleep at the wheel: Motor vehicle mishaps in persons taking pramipexole and ropinirole. *Neurology, 52*(9), 1908–1910.

Fujii, C., Harada, S., Ohkoshi, N., et al. (2000). Cross-cultural traits for personality of patients with Parkinson's disease in Japan. *American Journal of Medical Genetics, 96*, 1–3.

Fuster, J. M. (1989). *The prefrontal cortex*. New York: Raven Press.

Fuster, J. M. (2004). Upper processing stages of the perception-action cycle. *Trends in Cognitive Sciences, 8*, 143–145.

Fuster, J. M. (2008). *The prefrontal cortex* (4th ed.). Boston: Academic Press.

Gallagher, S. (2000). Philosophical conceptions of the self: Implications for cognitive science. *Trends in Cognitive Sciences, 4*(1), 14–21.

Gallese, V., Rochat, M., Cossu, G., & Sinigaglia, C. (2009). Motor cognition and its role in the phylogeny and ontogeny of action understanding. *Developmental Psychology, 45*(1), 103–113.

Gao, X., Simon, K. C., Han, J., Schwarzschild, M. A., & Ascherio, A. (2009). Genetic determinants of hair color and Parkinson's disease risk. *Annals of Neurology, 65*(1), 76–82.

Germain, A., & Nielsen, T. (2003). Impact of imagery rehearsal treatment on distressing dreams, psychological distress, and sleep parameters in nightmare patients. *Behavioral Sleep Medicine, 1*, 140–154.

German, D., Manaye, K., Smith, W., Woodward, D., & Saper, C. (1989). Mid-brain dopaminergic cell loss in Parkinson's disease: Computer visualization. *Annals of Neurology, 26*, 507–514.

Geschwind, N., & Galaburda, A. M. (1985a). Cerebral lateralization: Biological mechanisms, associations, and pathology: I. A hypothesis and a program for research. *Archives of Neurology, 42*, 428–459.

Geschwind, N., & Galaburda, A. M. (1985b). Cerebral lateralization: Biological mechanisms, associations, and pathology: II. A hypothesis and a program for research. *Archives of Neurology, 42*, 521–552.

Geschwind, N., & Galaburda, A. M. (1985c). Cerebral lateralization: Biological mechanisms, associations, and pathology: III. A hypothesis and a program for research. *Archives of Neurology, 42*, 634–654.

Geschwind, N., & Galaburda, A. M. (1987). *Cerebral lateralization: Biological mechanisms, associations and pathology*. Cambridge, MA: The MIT Press.

Geyer, J. L., & Grossman, M. (1994). Investigating the basis for the sentence comprehension deficits in Parkinson's disease. *Journal of Neurolinguistics, 8*(3), 191–205.

Gibb, W. R. G., & Lees, A. J. (1988). The relevance of the Lewy body to the pathogenesis of idiopathic Parkinson's disease. *Journal of Neurology, Neurosurgery, and Neuropsychiatry, 51*, 745–752.

Gibbs, R. W., Jr. (1999). *Intentions in the experience of meaning.* Cambridge, UK: Cambridge University Press.

Giedke, H., & Schwarzler, F. (2002). Therapeutic use of sleep deprivation in depression. *Sleep Medicine Reviews, 6,* 361–377.

Gildea, P., & Glucksberg, S. (1983). On understanding metaphor: The role of context. *Journal of Verbal Learning and Verbal Behavior, 22,* 577–590.

Gillin, J. C., Buchsbaum, M., Wu, J., Clark, C., & Bunney, W. (2001). Sleep deprivations as a model experimental antidepressant treatment: Findings from function brain imaging. *Depression and Anxiety, 14,* 37–49.

Global Parkinson's Disease Survey Steering Committee. (2002). Factors impacting on quality of life in Parkinson's disease: results from an international survey. *Movement Disorders, 17*(1), 60–67.

Glosser, G., Clark, C., Freundlich, B., Kliner-Krenzel, L., Flaherty, P., & Stern, M. (1995). A controlled investigation of current and premorbid personality: Characteristics of Parkinson's disease patients. *Movement Disorders, 10,* 201–206.

Glucksberg, S., Gildea, P., & Bookin, H. (1982). On understanding nonliteral speech: Can people ignore metaphors? *Journal of Verbal Learning and Verbal Behavior, 22,* 577–590.

Goetz, C. G. (2009). Jean-Martin Charcot and his vibratory chair for Parkinson disease. *Neurology, 73*(6), 475–478.

Goetz, C. G., & Stebbins, G. T. (1993). Risk factors for nursing home placement in advanced Parkinson's disease. *Neurology, 43*(11), 2227–2229.

Goetz, C. G., Leurgans, S., Pappert, E. J., Raman, R., & Stemer, A. B. (2001). Prospective longitudinal assessment of hallucinations in Parkinson's disease. *Neurology, 57*(11), 2078–2082.

Goetz, C. G., Tanner, C. M., Levy, M., Wilson, R. S., & Garron, D. C. (1986). Pain in Parkinson's disease. *Movement Disorders, 1*(1), 45–49.

Goetz, C. G., Tilley, B. C., Shaftman, S. R., Stebbins, G. T., Fahn, S., Martinez-Martin, P., et al. (2008). Movement Disorder Society-sponsored revision of the Unified Parkinson's Disease Rating Scale (MDS-UPDRS): Scale presentation and clinimetric testing results. *Movement Disorders, 23*(15), 2129–2170.

Goldman-Rakic, P. (1987). Circuitry of primate prefrontal cortex and regulation of behavior by representational memory. In V. Plum (Ed.), *Higher cortical function. Handbook of physiology* (pp. 373–417). New York: American Physiological Society.

Goldman-Rakic, P. S., Muly, E. C., & Williams, G. V. (2000). D(1) receptors in prefrontal cells and circuits. *Brain Research. Brain Research Reviews, 31*(2–3), 295–301.

Gollwitzer, P. M. (1990). Action phases and mind-sets. In E. T. Higgins & R. M. Sorrentino (Eds.), *The handbook of motivation and cognition: Foundations of social behavior* (Vol. 2, pp. 53–92). New York: Guilford Press.

Gollwitzer, P. M. (1993). Goal achievement: The role of intentions. *European Review of Social Psychology, 4,* 141–185.

Gollwitzer, P. M. (1999). Implementation intentions: Strong effects of simple plans. *American Psychologist, 54,* 493–503.

Gollwitzer, P. M., & Moskowitz, G. B. (1996). Goal effects on action and cognition. In E. T. Higgins & A. W. Kruglanski (Eds.), *Social psychology: Handbook of basic principles* (pp. 361–399). New York: Guilford Press.

Gollwitzer, P. M., & Schaal, B. (1998). Metacognition in action: The importance of implementation intentions. *Personality and Social Psychology Review, 2,* 124–136.

Goodenough, D. R. (1991). Dream recall: History and current status of the field. In S. J. Ellman & J. S. Antrobus (Eds.), *The mind in sleep: Psychology and psychophysiology* (2nd ed., pp. 143–171). New York: John Wiley & Sons.

Goodwin, G. M., Austin, M.-P., Dougall, N., Ross, M., Murray, C., O'Caroll, R. E., et al. (1993). State changes in brain activity shown by the uptake of ^{99m}Tc-exametazime with single photon emission tomography in major depression before and after treatment. *Journal of Affective Disorders, 29*(4), 243–253.

Goodwin, V. A., Richards, S. H., Taylor, R. S., Taylor, A. H., & Campbell, J. L. (2008). The effectiveness of exercise interventions for people with Parkinson's Disease: A systematic review and meta-analysis. *Movement Disorders, 23*(5), 631–640.

Gotham, A. M., Brown, R. G., & Marsden, C. D. (1988). 'Frontal' cognitive function in patients with Parkinson's disease 'on' and 'off' levodopa. *Brain, 111*, 299–321.

Gottesman, C., & Gottesman, I. (2007). The neurobiological characteristics of rapid eye movement (REM) sleep are candidate endophenotypes of depression, schizophrenia, mental retardation and dementia. *Progress in Neurobiology, 81*, 237–250.

Graboys, T., & Zheutlin, P. (2008). *Life in the balance: A physician's memoir of life, love and loss with Parkinson's disease and dementia.* New York: Union Square Press.

Grace, A. A. (1991). Phasic versus tonic dopamine release and the modulation of dopamine system responsivity: A hypothesis for the etiology of schizophrenia. *Neuroscience, 41*, 1–24.

Grace, A. A. (2002). Dopamine. In F. E. Bloom & D. J. Kupfer (Eds.), *Psychopharmacology, the fifth generation of progress* (pp. 119–132). Philadelphia: Lippincott Williams & Wilkins.

Gracey, F., Palmer, S., Rous, B., Psaila, K., Shaw, K., O'Dell, J., et al. (2008). "Feeling part of things": Personal construction of self after brain injury. *Neuropsychological Rehabilitation, 18*(5–6), 627–650.

Gregor, T. (2001). Content analysis of Mehinaku dreams. In K. Bulkeley (Ed.), *Dreams: A reader on the religious, cultural and psychological dimensions of dreaming* (pp. 133–166). New York: Palgrave.

Gregor, T. A. (1981). "Far far away my shadow wandered…" The dream theories of the Mehinaku Indians of Brazil. *American Ethnologist, 8*, 709–720.

Grice, H. P. (1975). Logic and conversation. In P. Cole & J. Morgan (Eds.), *Syntax and semantics, Vol. 3. Speech acts* (pp. 41–58). New York: Academic Press.

Grice, H. P. (1989). *Studies in the way of words.* Cambridge, MA: Harvard University Press.

Grossman, M., Carvell, S., Gollomp, S., Stern, M. B., Vernon, G., & Hurtig, H. I. (1991). Sentence comprehension and praxis deficits in Parkinson's disease. *Neurology, 41*, 1620–1626.

Grossman, M., Carvell, S., Stern, M. B., Gollomp, S., & Hurtig, H. I. (1992). Sentence comprehension in Parkinson's disease: The role of attention and memory. *Brain and Language, 42*, 347–384.

Grossman, M., Crino, P., Reivich, M., Stern, M. B., & Hurtig, H. I. (1992). Attention and sentence processing deficits in Parkinson's disease: The role of anterior cingulate cortex. *Cerebral Cortex, 2*, 513–525.

Grossman, M., Cooke, A., DeVita, C., Lee, C., Alsop, D., Detre, J., et al. (2003). Grammatical and resource components of sentence processing in Parkinson's disease: An fMRI study. *Neurology, 60*, 775–781.

Grossman, M., Glosser, G., Kalmanson, J., Morris, J., Stern, M. B., & Hurtig, H. I. (2001). Dopamine supports sentence comprehension in Parkinson's disease. *Journal of the Neurological Sciences, 184*(2), 123–130.

Grossman, M., Stern, M. B., Gollomp, S., Vernon, G., & Hurtig, H. I. (1994). Verb learning in Parkinson's disease. *Neuropsychology, 8*(3), 413–423.

Haaxma-Reiche, H., Piers, D. A., & Beekhuis, H. (1989). Normal cerebrospinal fluid dynamics: A study with intraventricular injection of 111In-DTPA in leukemia and lymphoma without meningeal involvement. *Archives of Neurology, 46*(9), 997–999.

Haggard, P., & Cole, J. (2007). Intention, attention and the temporal experience of action. *Consciousness and Cognition, 16*(2), 211–220.

Hairston, I. S., & Knight, R. T. (2004). Sleep on it. *Nature, 430*(6995), 27–28.

Happe, S., & Berger, K. (2002). The association between caregiver burden and sleep disturbances in partners of patients with Parkinson's disease. *Age and Ageing, 31*, 349–354.

Happe, S., Ludemann, P., & Berger, K. (2002). The association between disease severity and sleep-related problems in patients with Parkinson's disease. *Neuropsychobiology, 46*(2), 90–96.

Heberlein, I., Ludin, H.-P., Scholz, J., & Vieregge, P. (1998). Personality, depression, and premorbid lifestyle in twin pairs discordant for Parkinson's disease. *Journal of Neurology, Neurosurgery, and Psychiatry, 64*, 262–266.

Hely, M. A., Reid, W. G., Adena, M. A., Halliday, G. M., & Morris, J. G. (2008). The Sydney multicenter study of Parkinson's disease: The inevitability of dementia at 20 years. *Movement Disorders, 23*(6), 837–844.

Henry, J. D., & Crawford, J. R. (2004). Verbal fluency deficits in Parkinson's disease: A meta-analysis. *Journal of the International Neuropsychological Society, 10*, 608–623.

Hilker, R., Thomas, A. V., Klein, J. C., Weisenbach, S., Kalbe, E., Burghaus, S., et al. (2005). Dementia in Parkinson disease: Functional imaging of cholinergic and dopaminergic pathways. *Neurology, 65*, 1716–1722.

Hirano, S., Eckert, T., Flanagan, T., & Eidelberg, D. (2009). Metabolic networks for assessment of therapy and diagnosis in Parkinson's disease. *Movement Disorders, 24*, S725–S731.

Hobson, J. A., & Pace-Schott, E. F. (2002). The cognitive neuroscience of sleep: Neuronal systems, consciousness and learning. *Nature Reviews. Neuroscience, 3*(9), 679–693.

Hobson, J. A., Pace-Schott, E. F., & Stickgold, R. (2000). Dreaming and the brain: Toward a cognitive neuroscience of conscious states. *Behavioral and Brain Sciences, 23*(6), 793–842.

Hobson, J. A., Stickgold, R., & Pace-Schott, E. F. (1998). The neuropsychology of REM sleep dreaming. *Neuroreport, 9*, R1–R14.

Hochstadt, J., Nakano, H., Lieberman, P., & Friedman, J. (2006). The roles of sequencing and verbal working memory in sentence comprehension deficits in Parkinson's disease. *Brain and Language, 97*, 243–257.

Hoehn, M., & Yahr, M. (1967). Parkinsonism: Onset, progression, and mortality. *Neurology, 17*, 427–442.

Hollerman, J. R., & Schultz, W. (1998). Dopamine neurons report an error in the temporal prediction of reward during learning. *Nature Neuroscience, 1*, 304–309.

Holloway, R. L. (1968). The evolution of the primate brain: Some aspects of quantitative relations. *Brain Research, 7*, 121–172.

Holtgraves, T., & McNamara, P. (2010a). Pragmatic comprehension deficit in Parkinson's Disease. *Journal of Clinical and Experimental Neuropsychology, 32*(4), 388–397.

Holtgraves, T., & McNamara, P. (2010b). Parkinson's disease and politeness. *Journal of Language and Social Psychology, 29*(2), 178–193.

Holtgraves, T., McNamara, P., Cappaert, K., & Durso, R. (2010). Linguistic correlates of asymmetric motor symptom severity in Parkinson's disease. *Brain and Cognition, 72*(2), 189–196.

Hooker, C., Roese, N. J., & Park, S. (2000). Impoverished counterfactual thinking is associated with schizophrenia. *Psychiatry, 63*(4), 326–335.

Horowski, R., Horowski, L., Calne, S., & Calne, D. (2000). From Wilhelm von Humboldt to Hitler: Are prominent people more prone to have Parkinson's disease? *Parkinsonism & Related Disorders, 6*, 205–214.

Houk, J. C., Adams, J. L., & Barto, A. G. (1995). A model of how the basal ganglia generates and uses neural signals that predict reinforcement. In J. C. Houk, J. Davis, & D. Beiser (Eds.), *Models of information processing in the basal ganglia* (pp. 249–270). Cambridge, MA: The MIT Press.

Hoyle, R. H., & Sherrill, M. R. (2006). Future orientation in the self-system: Possible selves, self-regulation, and behavior. *Journal of Personality*, *74*, 1673–1696.

Hoyle, R. H., & Sowards, B. A. (1993). Self-monitoring and the regulation of social experience: A control-process model. *Journal of Social and Clinical Psychology*, *12*, 280–306.

Hubble, J. P., & Koller, W. C. (1995). The Parkinsonian personality. In W. J. Weiner & A. E. Lang (Eds.), *Behavioral neurology of movement disorders* (pp. 43–48). New York: Raven Press.

Hubble, J. P., Venkatesh, R., Hassanein, R. E., Gray, C., & Koller, W. C. (1993). Personality and depression in Parkinson's disease. *Journal of Nervous and Mental Disease*, *181*(11), 657–662.

Huber, R., Ghilardi, M. F., Massimini, M., & Tononi, G. (2004). Local sleep and learning. *Nature*, *430*, 78–81.

Hughes, A. J., Daniel, S. E., Kilford, L., & Lees, A. J. (1992). Accuracy of clinical diagnosis of idiopathic Parkinson's disease. A clinico-pathological study of 100 cases. *Journal of Neurology, Neurosurgery, and Neuropsychiatry*, *55*, 181–184.

Huttenlocher, P. R., & Dabholkar, A. S. (1997). Regional differences in synaptogenesis in human cerebral cortex. *Journal of Comparative Neurology*, *387*(2), 167–178.

Ibarretxe-Bilbao, N., Junque, C., Tolosa, E., Marti, M.-J., Valldeoriola, F., Bargallo, N., et al. (2009). Neuroanatomical correlates of impaired decision making and facial emotion recognition in early Parkinson's disease. *European Journal of Neuroscience*, *30*, 1162–1170.

Jacobs, D. M., Marder, K., Cote, L. J., Sano, M., Stern, Y., & Mayeux, R. (1995). Neuropsychological characteristics of preclinical dementia in Parkinson's disease. *Neurology*, *45*(9), 1691–1696.

Jacobs, H., Heberlein, I., Vieregge, A., & Vieregge, P. (2001). Personality traits in young patients with Parkinson's disease. *Acta Neurologica Scandinavica*, *103*(2), 82–87.

Janvin, C. C., Larsen, J. P., Salmon, D. P., Galasko, D., Hugdahl, K., & Aarsland, D. (2006). Cognitive profiles of individual patients with Parkinson's disease dementia: Comparison with dementia with Lewy bodies and Alzheimer's disease. *Movement Disorders*, *21*(3), 337–342.

Javoy-Agid, F., & Agid, Y. (1980). Is the mesocortical dopaminergic system involved in Parkinson's disease? *Neurology*, *30*, 1326–1330.

Jellinger, K. A., Seppi, K., Wenning, G. K., & Poewe, W. (2002). Impact of coexistent Alzheimer pathology on the natural history of Parkinson's disease. *Journal of Neural Transmission*, *109*(3), 329–339.

Jeannerod, M. (2004). Visual and action cues contribute to the self-other distinction. *Nature Neuroscience*, *7*(5), 422–423.

Jiménez-Jiménez, F. J., Santos, J., Zancada, F., Molina, J. A., Irastorza, J., Fernández-Ballesteros, A., et al. (1992). "Premorbid" personality of patients with Parkinson's disease. *Acta Neurologica*, *14*(3), 208–214.

Johnson, J. I. (1990). Comparative development of somatic sensory cortex. In E. G. Jones & A. Peters (Eds.), *Cerebral cortex* (pp. 335–449). New York: Plenum Press.

Johnson, P., & McNamara, P. (2007). Access to social action scripts in Parkinson's disease: Relation to side of onset. Poster presented at: UROP Symposium at Boston University; October 19, 2007; Boston, MA.

Jones, J. M. (2004). Great shakes: Famous people with Parkinson disease. *Southern Medical Association*, *97*(12), 1186–1189.

Jones, J. L., Day, J. J., Aragona, B. J., Wheeler, R. A., Wightman, R. M., & Carelli, R. M. (2010). Basolateral amygdala modulates terminal dopamine release in the nucleus accumbens and conditioned responding. *Biological Psychiatry*, *67*(8), 737–744.

Josephs, I. E., & Ribbert, H. (2003). Where is the other in the self? In M. Brüne, H. Ribber, & W. Schiefenhovel (Eds.), *The social brain: Evolution and pathology* (pp. 153–166). Chichester, UK: Wiley.

Juyal, R., Das, M., Punia, S., Madhuri, B., Nainway, G., Singh, S., et al. (2006). Genetic susceptibility to Parkinson's disease among South and North Indians: I. Role of polymorphisms in dopamine receptor and transporter genes and association of DRD4 120-bp duplication marker. *Neurogenetics*, *7*, 223–229.

Kaasinen, V., Nurmi, E., Bergman, J., Eskola, O., Solin, O., Sonninen, P., et al. (2001). Personality traits and brain dopaminergic function in Parkinson's disease. *Proceedings of the National Academy of Sciences of the United States of America*, *98*(23), 13272–13277.

Kahneman, D. (2003). A perspective on judgment and choice: Mapping bounded rationality. *American Psychologist*, *58*, 697–720.

Kahneman, D., & Miller, D. T. (1986). Norm theory: Comparing reality to its alternatives. *Psychological Review*, *93*, 136–153.

Kahneman, D., & Tversky, A. (1979). Prospect theory: An analysis of decision under risk. *Econometrica*, *47*(2), 263–292.

Kan, Y., Kawamura, M., Hasegawa, Y., Mochizuki, S., & Nakamura, K. (2002). Recognition of emotion from facial, prosodic and written verbal stimuli in Parkinson's disease. *Cortex*, *38*, 623–630.

Karlsen, K., Larsen, J. P., Tandberg, E., & Jorgensen, K. (1999). Fatigue in patients with Parkinson's disease. *Movement Disorders*, *14*(2), 237–241.

Katai, S., Maruyama, T., Hashimoto, T., & Ikeda, S. (2003). Event based and time based prospective memory in Parkinson's disease. *Journal of Neurology, Neurosurgery, and Psychiatry*, *74*(6), 704–709.

Kennedy, S. H., Evans, K. R., Kruger, S., Mayberg, H. S., Meyer, J. H., McCann, S., et al. (2001). Changes in regional brain glucose metabolism measured with positron emission tomography after paroxetine treatment of major depression. *American Journal of Psychiatry*, *158*, 899–905.

Kemmerer, D. (1999). Impaired comprehension of raising-to-subject constructions in Parkinson's disease. *Brain and Language*, *66*, 311–328.

Keysar, B. (1989). On the functional equivalence of literal and metaphorical interpretation in discourse. *Journal of Memory and Language*, *28*, 375–385.

Keysers, C., & Gazzola, V. (2007). Integrating simulation and theory of mind: From self to social cognition. *Trends in Cognitive Sciences*, *11*(5), 194–196.

Kieling, C., Roman, T., Doyle, A., Hutz, M., & Rohde, L. (2006). Association between DRD4 gene and performance of children with ADHD in a test of sustained attention. *Biological Psychiatry*, *60*, 1163–1165.

Kirsch-Darrow, L., Fernandez, H. F., Marsiske, M., Okun, M. S., & Bowers, D. (2006). Dissociating apathy and depression in Parkinson disease. *Neurology*, *67*, 33–38.

Kliegel, M., Phillips, L. H., Lemke, U., & Kopp, U. A. (2005). Planning and realisation of complex intentions in patients with Parkinson's disease. *Journal of Neurology, Neurosurgery, and Psychiatry*, *76*, 1501–1505.

Knutson, B., & Bhanji, J. (2006). Neural substrates for emotional traits: The case of extraversion. In T. Canli (Ed.), *Biology of personality and individual differences* (pp. 116–132). New York: The Guilford Press.

Kobayakawa, M., Koyama, S., Mumura, M., & Kawamura, M. (2008). Decision making in Parkinson's disease: Analysis of behavioral and physiological patterns in the Iowa gambling task. *Movement Disorders*, *23*, 547–552.

Koechlin, E., & Summerfield, C. (2007). An information theoretical approach to prefrontal executive function. *Trends in Cognitive Sciences*, *11*, 229–235.

Koenigs, M., Huey, E., Calamia, M., Raymont, V., Tranel, D., & Grafman, J. (2008). Distinct regions of prefrontal cortex mediate resistance and vulnerability to depression. *Journal of Neuroscience*, *28*, 12341–12348.

Kondracke, M. (2001). *Saving Milly. Love, politics, and Parkinson's disease*. Cambridge, MA: The Perseus Books Group.

Korf, J., Grasdijk, L., & Westerink, B. H. C. (1976). Effects of electrical stimulation of the nigrostriatal pathway of the rat on dopamine metabolism. *Journal of Neurochemistry*, *26*, 579.

Kramer, M. (1993). The selective mood regulatory function of dreaming: An update and revision. In A. Moffit, M. Kramer, & R. Hoffman (Eds.), *The functions of dreaming* (pp. 139–196). Albany, NY: State University of New York Press.

Kronenberg, M. F., Menzel, H. J., Ebersbach, G., Wenning, G. K., Luginger, E., Gollner, M., et al. (1999). Dopamine D4 receptor polymorphism and idiopathic Parkinson's disease. *European Journal of Human Genetics*, *7*(3), 397–400.

Kuiken, D., & Sikora, S. (1993). The impact of dreams on waking thoughts and feelings. In A. Moffitt, M. Kramer, & R. Hoffman (Eds.), *The functions of dreaming* (pp. 419–476). Albany, NY: State University of New York Press.

Kuiper, M. A., & Wolters, E. Ch. (1995). CSF biochemistry in Parkinson's disease patients with mental dysfunction. In E. Wolters & P. Scheltens (Eds.), *Mental dysfunction in Parkinson's disease* (pp. 163–176). Dordrecht, The Netherlands: ICG.

Kulisevsky, J., Asuncion, A., Barbanoj, M., Antonijoan, R., Berthier, M. L., Gironell, A., et al. (1996). Acute effects of levodopa on neuropsychological performance in stable and fluctuating Parkinson's disease patients at different levodopa plasma levels. *Brain*, *119*(6), 2121–2132.

Kulisevsky, J., & Pagonabarraga, J. (2010). Cognitive impairment in Parkinson's disease: Tools for diagnosis and assessment. *Movement Disorders*, *24*(8), 1103–1110.

Kulisevsky, J., Pagonabarraga, J., Pascual-Sedano, B., Garcia-Sanchez, C., & Gironell, A. (2008). Prevalence and correlates of neuropsychiatric symptoms in Parkinson's disease without dementia. *Movement Disorders*, *23*(13), 1889–1896.

Kumar, S., Bhatia, M., & Behari, M. (2002). Sleep disorders in Parkinson's disease. *Movement Disorders*, *17*(4), 775–781.

Kupfer, D. J., & Foster, G. (1972). Interval between onset of sleep and rapid-eye-movement sleep as an indicator of depression. *Lancet*, *2*, 684–686.

Lange, K. W., Paul, G. M., Naumann, M., & Gesell, W. (1995). Dopaminergic effects on cognitive performance in patients with Parkinson's disease. *Journal of Neural Transmission*, *46*(Suppl), 423–432.

Lange, K. W., Paul, G. M., Robbins, T. W., & Marsden, C. D. (1993). L-dopa and frontal cognitive function in Parkinson's disease. In H. Narabayashi, T. Nagatsu, N. Yanagisawa, & Y. Mizuno (Eds.), *Advances in neurology* (Vol. 60, pp. 475–478). New York: Raven Press, Ltd.

Lange, K. W., Robbins, T. W., Marsden, C. D., James, M., Owen, A. M., & Paul, G. M. (1992). L-dopa withdrawal in Parkinson's disease selectively impairs cognitive performance in tests sensitive to frontal lobe dysfunction. *Psychopharmacology*, *107*, 394–404.

Larsen, J. P., & Tandberg, E. (2001). Sleep disorders in patients with Parkinson's disease: Epidemiology and management. *CNS Drugs*, *15*(4), 267–275.

Laureys, S., Peigneux, P., Phillips, C., Fuchs, S., Degueldre, C., Aerts, J., et al. (2001). Experience-dependent changes in cerebral functional connectivity during rapid eye movement sleep. *Neuroscience*, *105*, 521–525.

Lauterbach, E. C. (2005). The neuropsychiatry of Parkinson's disease. *Minerva Medica*, *96*(3), 155–173.

Ledoux, J. (2000). The amygdala and emotion: A view through fear. In J. P. Aggleton (Ed.), *The amygdala: A functional analysis* (pp. 289–310). Oxford, UK: Oxford University Press.

Lees, A. J., & Smith, E. (1983). Cognitive deficits in the early stages of Parkinson's disease. *Brain*, *106*, 257–270.

Lees, A. J., Blackburn, N. A., & Campbell, V. L. (1988). The nighttime problems of Parkinson's disease. *Clinical Neuropharmacology*, *11*(6), 512–519.

Lemke, M. R. (2002). Effect of reboxetine on depression in Parkinson's disease patients. *Journal of Clinical Psychiatry*, *63*, 300–304.

Leube, D. T., Knoblich, G., Erb, M., Grodd, W., Bartels, M., & Kircher, T. T. (2003). The neural correlates of perceiving one's own movements. *NeuroImage, 20*(4), 2084–2090.

Levin, B. E., Llabre, M. M., & Weiner, W. J. (1989). Cognitive impairments associated with early Parkinson's disease. *Neurology, 39*(4), 557–561.

Levy, R., & Dubois, B. (2006). Apathy and the functional anatomy of the prefrontal cortex-basal ganglia circuits. *Cerebral Cortex, 16*, 916–928.

Levy, M. L., Cummings, J. L., Fairbanks, L. A., Masterman, D., Miller, B. L., Craig, A. H., et al. (1998). Apathy is not depression. *Journal of Neuropsychiatry, 10*(3), 314–319.

Levy, G., Jacobs, D. M., Tang, M. X., Cote, L. J., Louis, E. D., Alfaro, B., et al. (2002). Memory and executive function impairment predict dementia in Parkinson's disease. *Movement Disorders, 17*(6), 1221–1226.

Lewis, D. A., Campbell, M. J., Foote, S. L., & Morrison, J. H. (1986). The monoaminergic innervations of primate neocortex. *Human Neurobiology, 5*, 181–188.

Lewis, S. J. G., Slabosz, A., Robbins, T. W., Barker, R. A., & Owen, A. M. (2005). Dopaminergic basis for deficits in working memory but not in attentional set-shifting in Parkinson's disease. *Neuropsychologia, 43*, 823–832.

Leyton, M., Boileau, I., Benkelfat, C., Diksic, M., Baker, G., & Dagher, A. (2002). Amphetamine-induced increases in extracellular dopamine, drug wanting, and novelty seeking: A PET/[11C]raclopride study in healthy men. *Neuropsychopharmacology, 27*, 1027–1035.

Libet, B. (1985). Unconscious cerebral initiative and the role of conscious will in voluntary action. *Behavioral and Brain Sciences, 8*, 529–566.

Lidow, M. S., Goldman-Rakic, P. S., Gallagpher, D. V., & Rakic, P. (1991). Distribution of dopaminergic receptors in the primate cerebral cortex: Quantitative autoradiographic analysis using [3H] raclopride, [3H] spiperone and [3H] SCH 23390. *Neuroscience, 40*, 657–671.

Lieberman, M. D. (2007). Social cognitive neuroscience: A review of core processes. *Annual Review of Psychology, 58*, 259–289.

Lieberman, P., Friedman, J., & Feldman, L. S. (1990). Syntax comprehension deficits in Parkinson's disease. *Journal of Nervous and Mental Disease, 178*, 360–365.

Lieberman, P., Kako, E., Friedman, J., Tajchman, G., Feldman, L. S., & Jiminez, E. B. (1992). Speech production, syntax comprehension and cognitive deficits in Parkinson's disease. *Brain and Language, 43*, 169–189.

Liotta, M., Mayberg, H. S., Brannan, S. K., McGinnis, S., Jerabek, P., & Fox, P. T. (2000). Differentials corticolimbic correlates of sadness and anxiety in healthy subjects: Implications for affective disorders. *Biological Psychiatry, 48*, 30–42.

Litvan, I., Mohr, E., Williams, J., Gomez, C., & Chase, T. N. (1991). Differential memory and executive functions in demented patients with Parkinson's and Alzheimer's disease. *Journal of Neurology, Neurosurgery, and Psychiatry, 54*, 25–29.

Longworth, C. E., Keenan, S. E., Barker, R. A., Marslen-Wilson, W. D., & Tyler, L. K. (2005). The basal ganglia and rule-governed language use: Evidence from vascular and degenerative conditions. *Brain, 128*, 584–596.

Loomes, G., & Sugden, R. (1982). Regret theory: An alternative theory of rational choice under uncertainty. *Economic Journal, 92*, 805–824.

Lovibond, S. H., & Lovibond, P. F. (1995). *Manual for the Depression Anxiety Stress Scales.* Sydney, Australia: The Psychology Foundation of Australia.

Machover, S. (1957). Rorschach study on the nature and origin of common factors in the personalities of Parkinsonians. *Psychosomatic Medicine, 19*(4), 332–338.

Marder, K. (2010). Cognitive impairment and dementia in Parkinson's disease. *Movement Disorders, 25*(Suppl. 1), S110–S116.

Markus, H., & Kunda, Z. (1986). Stability and malleability in the self-concept in the perception of others. *Journal of Personality and Social Psychology, 51*(4), 858–866.

Markus, H., & Nurius, P. (1986). Possible selves. *American Psychologist, 41*, 954–969.

Maquet, P., & Franck, G. (1997). REM sleep and amygdala. *Molecular Psychiatry, 2*(3), 195–196.

Maquet, P., Peters, J.-M., Aerts, J., Delfiore, G., Degueldre, C., Luxen, A., et al. (1996). Functional neuro-anatomy of human rapid-eye-movement sleep and dreaming. *Nature, 383*, 163–166.

Maquet, P., Ruby, P., Maudoux, A., Albouy, G., Sterpenich, V., Dang-Vu, T., et al. (2005). Human cognition during REM sleep and the activity profile within frontal and parietal cortices: A reappraisal of functional neuroimaging data. *Progress in Brain Research, 150*, 219–227.

Maquet, P., Smith, C., & Stickgold, R. (Eds.). (2003). *Sleep and plasticity.* New York: Oxford University Press.

Marin, R. S. (1996). Apathy: Concept, syndrome, neural mechanisms, and treatment. *Seminars in Clinical Neuropsychiatry, 1*(4), 304–314.

Marsh, L., Williams, J. R., Rocco, M., Grill, S., Munro, C., & Dawson, T. M. (2004). Psychiatric comorbidities in patients with Parkinson disease and psychosis. *Neurology, 63*(2), 293–300.

Massimi, M., Berry, E., Browne, G., Smyth, G., Waton, P., & Baecker, R. M. (2008). An exploratory case study of the impact of ambient biographical displays on identity in a patient with Alzheimer's disease. *Neuropsychological Rehabilitation, 18*(5–6), 742–765.

Mathias, J. L. (2003). Neurobehavioral functioning of persons with Parkinson's disease. *Applied Neuropsychology, 10*(2), 57–68.

Mattay, V. S., Callicott, J. H., Bertolino, A., Heaton, I., Frank, J. A., Coppola, R., et al. (2000). Effects of dextroamphetamine on cognitive performance and cortical activation. *NeuroImage, 12*, 268–275.

Mattay, V. S., Tessitore, A., Callicott, J. H., Bertolino, A., Goldberg, T. E., Chase, T. N., et al. (2002). Dopaminergic modulation of cortical function in patients with Parkinson's disease. *Annals of Neurology, 51*, 156–164.

Mayberg, H. S. (1994). Frontal lobe dysfunction in secondary depression. *Journal of Neuropsychiatry and Clinical Neurosciences, 6*, 428–442.

Mayberg, H. S., Brannan, S. K., Mahurin, R. K., Jerabek, P. A., Brickman, J. S., Tekell, J. L., et al. (1997). Cingulate function in depression: A potential predictor of treatment response. *Neuroreport, 8*(4), 1057–1061.

Mayberg, H. S., Brannan, S. K., Tekell, J. L., Silva, J. A., Mahurin, R. K., McGinnis, S., et al. (2000). Regional metabolic effects of fluoxetine in major depression: Serial changes and relationship to clinical response. *Biological Psychiatry, 48*, 830–843.

Mayberg, H. S., Liotti, M., Brannan, S. K., McGinnis, S., Mahurin, R. K., Jerabek, P. A., et al. (1999). Reciprocal limbic-cortical function and negative mood: Converging PET findings in depression and normal sadness. *American Journal of Psychiatry, 156*, 675–682.

McDaniel, M. A., & Einstein, G. O. (2007). *Prospective memory: An overview and synthesis of an emerging field.* Thousand Oaks, CA: Sage.

McKeith, I. G., Dickson, D. W., Lowe, J., Emre, M., O'Brien, J. T., Feldman, H., et al. (2005). Diagnosis and management of dementia with Lewy bodies. *Neurology, 65*, 1863–1872.

McNamara, P. (2008). *Nightmares: The science and solution of those frightening visions during sleep.* Westport, CT: Praeger.

McNamara, P. (2009). *The neuroscience of religious experience.* New York: Cambridge University Press.

McNamara, P., & Durso, R. (1991). Reversible Othello syndrome in a man with Parkinson's disease. *American Journal of Geriatric Neurology and Psychiatry, 4*(3), 157–159.

McNamara, P., & Durso, R. (2000). Language functions in Parkinson's disease: Evidence for a neuro-chemistry of language. In L. Obler & L. T. Connor (Eds.), *Neurobehavior of language and cognition: Studies of normal aging and brain damage* (pp. 201–212). New York: Kluwer Academic Publishers.

McNamara, P., & Durso, R. (2003). Pragmatic communication skills in patients with Parkinson's disease. *Brain and Language, 84*, 414–423.

McNamara, P., Clark, J., Krueger, M., & Durso, R. (1996). Grammaticality judgments and sentence comprehension in Parkinson's disease: A comparison with Broca's aphasia. *International Journal of Neuroscience, 86*, 151–166.

McNamara, P., Durso, R., & Brown, A. (2003). Relation of 'sense of self' to executive function performance in Parkinson's disease. *Cognitive and Behavioral Neurology, 14*, 139–148.

McNamara, P., Durso, R., Brown, A., & Lynch, A. (2003). Counterfactual cognitive deficit in patients with Parkinson's disease. *Journal of Neurology, Neurosurgery, and Psychiatry, 74*, 1065–1070.

McNamara, P., Durso, R., & Harris, E. (2006a). Life goals of patients with Parkinson's disease: A pilot study on correlations with mood and cognitive functions. *Clinical Rehabilitation, 20*, 818–826.

McNamara, P., Durso, R., & Harris, E. (2006b). Frontal lobe mediation of the sense of self: Evidence from studies of patients with Parkinson's disease. In A. P. Prescott (Ed.), *The concept of self in medicine and health care* (pp. 143–161). Hauppauge, NY: Nova Science Publishers, Inc.

McNamara, P., Durso, R., & Harris, E. (2007). "Machiavellianism" and frontal dysfunction: Evidence from Parkinson's disease (PD). *Cognitive Neuropsychiatry, 12*(4), 285–300.

McNamara, P., Durso, R., & Harris, E. (2008). Alterations of the sense of self and personality in Parkinson's disease. *International Journal of Geriatric Psychiatry, 23*(1), 79–84.

McNamara, P., Holtgraves, T., Durso, R., & Harris, E. (2010). Social cognition of indirect speech: Evidence from Parkinson's disease. *Journal of Neurolinguistics, 23*(2), 162–171.

McNamara, P., Johnson, P., McLaren, D., Harris, E., Beauharnais, C., & Auerbach, S. (2010). REM and NREM sleep mentation. *International Review of Neurobiology. 92*, 69–86.

McNamara, P., McLaren, D., & Durso, K. (2007). Representation of the self in REM and NREM dreams. *Dreaming, 17*(2), 113–126.

McNamara, P., McLaren, D., Smith, D., Brown, A., & Stickgold, R. (2005). A "Jekyll and Hyde" within: Aggressive versus friendly social interactions in REM and NREM dreams. *Psychological Science, 16*(2), 130–136.

McNamara, P., Obler, L. K., Au, R., Durso, R., & Albert, M. (1992). Speech monitoring skills in Alzheimer's disease, Parkinson's disease and normal aging. *Brain and Language, 42*, 38–51.

McNamara, P., Stavitsky, K., Harris, E., Szent-Imrey, O., & Durso, R. (2010). Mood, side of motor symptom onset and pain complaints in Parkinson's disease. *International Journal of Geriatric Psychiatry, 25*(5), 519–524.

Mead, G. H. (1934). *Mind, self and society*. Chicago: University of Chicago Press.

Mendelsohn, G. A., Dakof, G. A., & Skaff, M. (1995). Personality change in Parkinson's disease patients: Chronic disease and aging. *Journal of Personality, 63*, 233–257.

Mengelberg, A., & Siegert, R. J. (2003). Is theory-of-mind impaired in Parkinson's disease? *Cognitive Neuropsychiatry, 8*(3), 191–209.

Melzack, R. (1975). The McGill Pain Questionnaire: Major properties and scoring methods. *Pain, 1*, 277–299.

Menza, M. A., Sage, J., Marshall, E., et al. (1990). Mood changes and 'on–off' phenomena in Parkinson's disease. *Movement Disorders, 5*, 148–151.

Menza, M. A., Golbe, L. I., Cody, R. A., & Forman, N. E. (1993). Dopamine-related personality traits in Parkinson's disease. *Neurology, 43*, 505–508.

Menza, M. A., Mark, M. H., Burn, D. J., & Brooks, D. J. (1995). Personality correlates of [18F]dopa striatal updated: Results of positron-emission tomography in Parkinson's disease. *Journal of Neuropsychiatry and Clinical Neurosciences, 7*(2), 176–179.

Metzinger, T. (2003). *Being no one: The self-model theory of subjectivity.* Cambridge, MA: The MIT Press.

Mimura, M., Oeda, R., & Kawamura, M. (2006). Impaired decision-making in Parkinson's disease. *Parkinsonism & Related Disorders, 12,* 169–175.

Monetta, L., Grindrod, C. M., & Pell, M. D. (2009). Irony comprehension and theory of mind deficits in patients with Parkinson's disease. *Cortex, 45*(8), 972–981.

Montague, P. R., Dayan, P., & Sejnowski, T. J. (1996). A framework for mesencephalic dopamine systems based on predictive Hebbian learning. *Journal of Neuroscience, 76*(5), 1936–1947.

Montplaisir, J., Nicolas, A., Godbout, R., & Walters, A. (2000). Restless leg syndrome and periodic limb movement disorders. In M. H. Kryger, T. Roth, & W. C. Dement (Eds.), *Principles and practice of sleep medicine* (3rd ed., pp. 742–752). Philadelphia: W. B. Saunders.

Morris, R. G., Downes, J. J., Sahakian, B. J., Evenden, J. L., Heald, A., & Robbins, T. W. (1988). Planning and spatial working memory in Parkinson's disease. *Journal of Neurology, Neurosurgery, and Psychiatry, 51*(6), 757–766. http://www.ninds.nih.gov/research/clinical_research/rfi.htm.

Natsopoulos, D., Grouios, G., Bostantzopoulou, S., Mentenopoulos, G., Katsarou, Z., & Logothetis, J. (1993). Algorithmic and heuristic strategies in comprehension of complement clauses by patients with Parkinson's disease. *Neuropsychologia, 31*(9), 951–964.

Natsopoulos, D., Katsarou, Z., Bostantzopoulou, S., Grouios, G., Mentenopoulos, G., & Logothetis, J. (1991). Strategies in comprehension of relative clauses by Parkinsonian patients. *Cortex, 27,* 255–268.

Naylor, E., & Clare, L. (2008). Awareness of memory functioning, autobiographical memory and identity in early-stage dementia. *Neuropsychological Rehabilitation, 18*(5–6), 590–606.

Niv, Y., Daw, N. D., Joel, D., & Dayan, P. (2007). Tonic dopamine: Opportunity costs and the control of response vigor. *Psychopharmacology, 191,* 507–520.

Nobili, F., Campus, C., Arnaldi, D., De Carli, F., Cabassi, G., Brugnolo, A., et al. (2010). Cognitive-nigrostriatal relationships in de novo, drug-naïve Parkinson's disease patients: A [I-123]FP-CIT SPECT study. *Movement Disorders, 25,* 35–43.

Noe, E., Marder, K., Bell, K. L., Jacobs, D. M., Manly, J. J., & Stern, Y. (2004). Comparison of dementia with Lewy bodies to Alzheimer's disease and Parkinson's disease with dementia. *Movement Disorders, 19,* 60–67.

Nofzinger, E. A. (2008). Functional neuroimaging of sleep disorders. *Current Pharmaceutical Design, 14*(32), 3417–3429.

Nofzinger, E. A., & Keshavan, M. (2002). Sleep disturbances associated with neuropsychiatric disease. In D. Charney, J. Coyle, K. Davis, & C. Nemeroff (Eds.), *American College of Neuropsychopharmacology: The fifth generation of progress* (pp. 1945–1959). Philadelphia: Lippincott Williams & Wilkins.

Nofzinger, E. A., Berman, S., Fasiczka, A., Miewald, J. M., Meltzer, C. C., Price, J. C., et al. (2001). Effects of bupropion SR on anterior paralimbic function during waking and REM sleep in depression: Preliminary findings using. *Psychiatry Research, 106*(2), 95–111.

Nofzinger, E. A., Buysse, D. J., Germain, A., Carter, C., Luna, B., Price, J. C., et al. (2004). Increased activation of anterior paralimbic and executive cortex from waking to rapid eye movement sleep in depression. *Archives of General Psychiatry, 61*(7), 695–702.

Nofzinger, E. A., Mintun, M. A., Wiseman, M. B., Kupfer, D. J., & Moore, R. Y. (1997). Forebrain activation in REM sleep: An FDG PET study. *Brain Research, 770,* 192–201.

Nofzinger, E. A., Nichols, T. E., Meltzer, C. C., Price, J., Steppe, D. A., Miewald, J. M., et al. (1999). Changes in forebrain function from waking to REM sleep in depression preliminary analyses of (18F) FDG PET studies. *Psychiatry Research*, *91*(2), 59–78.

Norman, C. C., & Aron, A. (2003). Aspects of possible self that predict motivation to achieve or avoid it. *Journal of Experimental Social Psychology*, *39*, 500–507.

Northoff, G., & Bermpohl, F. (2004). Cortical midline structures and the self. *Trends in Cognitive Sciences*, *8*, 102–107.

Nutt, D. J., Wilson, S. J., & Paterson, L. M. (2008). Sleep disorders as core symptoms of depression. *Dialogues in Clinical Neuroscience*, *10*, 329–335.

Oades, R. D., & Halliday, G. M. (1987). Ventral tegmental (A10) system: Neurobiology: 1. Anatomy and connectivity. *Brain Research*, *434*, 117–165.

Oatley, K. (2007). Narrative modes of consciousness and selfhood. In P. D. Zelazo, M. Moscovitch, & E. Thompson (Eds.), *The Cambridge handbook of consciousness* (pp. 375–402). New York: Cambridge. University Press.

Ochsner, K. N., Ray, R. D., Cooper, J. C., Robertson, E. R., Chopra, S., Gabrieli, J. D., et al. (2004). For better or for worse: Neural systems supporting the cognitive down- and up-regulation of negative emotion. *NeuroImage*, *23*, 483–499.

Oguru, M., Tachibana, H., Toda, K., Okuda, B., & Oka, N. (2010). Apathy and depression in Parkinson disease. *Journal of Geriatric Psychiatry and Neurology*, *23*(1), 35–41.

Oldenhof, J., Vickery, R., Anafi, M., Oak, J., Ray, A., Schoots, O., et al. (1998). SH3-binding domains in the dopamine D4 receptor. *Biochemistry*, *37*, 15726–15736.

Olson, E. J., Boeve, B. F., & Silber, M. H. (2000). Rapid eye movement sleep behaviour disorder: Demographic, clinical and laboratory findings in 93 cases. *Brain*, *123*(Pt 2), 331–339.

Onofrj, M., Thomas, A., D'Andreamatteo, G., Iacono, D., Luciano, A. L., Di Rollo, A., et al. (2002). Incidence of RBD and hallucination in patients affected by Parkinson's disease: 8-year follow-up. *Neurological Sciences*, *23*(Suppl. 2), S91–S94.

Owen, A. M. (2004). Cognitive dysfunction in Parkinson's disease: The role of frontostriatal circuitry. *Neuroscientist*, *10*(6), 525–537.

Owen, A. M., James, M., Leigh, P. N., Summers, B. A., Marsden, C. D., Quinn, N. P., et al. (1992). Frontostriatal cognitive deficits at different stages of Parkinson's disease. *Brain*, *115*(6), 1727–1751.

Oyserman, D., Bybee, D., Terry, K., & Hart-Johnson, T. (2004). Possible selves as roadmaps. *Journal of Research in Personality*, *38*, 130–149.

Pace-Schott, E. F. (2007). The frontal lobes and dreaming. In D. Barrett & P. McNamara (Eds.), *The new science of dreaming, Vol. 1: Biological aspects* (pp. 115–154). Westport, CT: Praeger.

Pagonabarraga, J., Garcia-Sanchez, C., Llebaria, G., Pascual-Sedano, B., Grionell, A., & Kulisevsky, J. (2007). Controlled study of decision-making and cognitive impairment in Parkinson's disease. *Movement Disorders*, *22*, 1430–1435.

Pal, P. K., Calne, S., Samii, A., & Fleming, J. A. E. (1999). A review of normal sleep and its disturbances in Parkinson's disease. *Parkinsonism & Related Disorders*, *5*, 1–17.

Pandya, D. N., & Seltzer, B. (1982). Intrinsic connections and architectonics of posterior parietal cortex in the rhesus monkey. *Journal of Comparative Neurology*, *204*, 196–210.

Pandya, D. N., Seltzer, B., & Barbas, H. (1988). Input-output organization of the primate cerebral cortex. In H. D. Steklis & J. Erwin (Eds.), *Comparative primate biology, Vol. 4, Neurosciences* (pp. 39–80). New York: Alan R. Liss.

Pappert, E. J., Goetz, C. G., Niederman, F. G., Raman, R., & Leurgans, S. (1999). Hallucinations, sleep fragmentation, and altered dream phenomena in Parkinson's disease. *Movement Disorders*, *14*(1), 117–121.

Parkinson, J. (1917). *An essay on the shaking palsy*. London, UK: Sherwood, Neeley, Jones.

Partinen, M. (1997). Sleep disorder related to Parkinson's disease. *Journal of Neurology, 244* (4, Suppl. 1), S3–S6.

Passingham, R. (1973). Anatomical differences between the neocortex of man and other primates. *Brain, Behavior and Evolution, 7*, 337–359.

Passingham, R. (1993). *The frontal lobes and voluntary action*. Oxford, UK: Oxford University Press.

Passingham, R. E., & Ettlinger, G. (1974). A comparison of cortical functions in man and the other primates. *International Review of Neurobiology, 16*, 233–299.

Paus, S., Seeger, G., Brecht, H., Koster, J., El-Faddagh, M., Nothen, M., et al. (2004). Association study of dopamine D2, D3, D4 receptor and serotonin transporter gene polymorphisms with sleep attacks in Parkinson's disease. *Movement Disorders, 19*(6), 705–707.

Pedersen, K. F., Alves, G., Aarsland, D., & Larsen, J. P. (2009). Occurrence and risk factors for apathy in Parkinson disease: A 4-year prospective longitudinal study. *Journal of Neurology, Neurosurgery, and Psychiatry, 80*, 1279–1282.

Penke, L., Denissen, J. J. A., & Miller, G. F. (2007). The evolutionary genetics of personality. *European Journal of Personality, 21*, 549–587.

Pennebaker, J. W., Booth, R. J., & Francis, M. E. (2007). *Linguistic Inquiry and Word Count (LIWC): LIWC, 2007*. Available at <http://www.liwc.net>.

Péron, J., Vicente, S., Leray, E., Drapier, S., Drapier, D., Cohen, R., et al. (2009). Are dopaminergic pathways involved in theory of mind? A study in Parkinson's disease. *Neuropsychologia, 47*(2), 406–414.

Perretta, J. G., Pari, G., & Beninger, R. J. (2005). Effects of Parkinson disease on two putative nondeclarative learning tasks: Probabilistic classification and gambling. *Cognitive and Behavioral Neurology, 18*, 185–192.

Petrides, M., & Pandya, D. N. (1999). Dorsolateral prefrontal cortex: Comparative cytoarchitectonic analysis in the human and the macaque brain and corticocortical connection patterns. *European Journal of Neuroscience, 11*(3), 1011–1036.

Piccirilli, M., D'Alessandro, P., Finali, G., Piccinin, G. L., & Agostini, L. (1989). Frontal lobe dysfunction in Parkinson's disease: Prognostic value for dementia? *European Neurology, 29*(2), 71–76.

Pillon, B., Deweer, B., Agid, Y., & Dubois, B. (1993). Explicit memory in Alzheimer's, Huntington's and Parkinson's diseases. *Archives of Neurology, 50*, 374–379.

Pine, A., Shiner, T., Seymour, B., & Dolan, R. J. (2010). Dopamine, time, and impulsivity in humans. *Journal of Neuroscience, 30*(26), 8888–8896.

Plihal, W., & Born, J. (1997). Effects of early and late nocturnal sleep on declarative and procedural memory. *Journal of Cognitive Neuroscience, 9*, 534–547.

Pluck, G. C., & Brown, R. G. (2002). Apathy in Parkinson's disease. *Journal of Neurology, Neurosurgery, and Psychiatry, 73*, 636–642.

Poewe, W., Karamat, E., Kemmler, G. W., & Gerstenbrand, F. (1990). The premorbid personality of patients with Parkinson's disease: A comparative study with healthy controls and patients with essential tremor. *Advances in Neurology, 53*, 339–342.

Poewe, W., Wolters, E., Emre, M., Onofrj, M., Hsu, C., Tekin, S., et al. (2006). Long-term benefits of rivastigmine in dementia associated with Parkinson's disease: An active treatment extension study. *Movement Disorders, 21*(4), 456–461.

Poletti, M., Frosini, D., Lucetti, C., Del Dotto, P., Ceravolo, R., & Bonuccelli, U. (2010). Decision making in de novo Parkinson's disease. *Movement Disorders, 25*(10), 1432–1436.

Post, R. M., Kotin, J., & Goodwin, F. K. (1973). Psychomotor activity and CSF amine metabolites in affective illness. *American Journal of Psychiatry, 130*, 67–72.

Preuss, T. M. (1995). Do rats have prefrontal cortex? The Rose-Woolsey-Akert program reconsidered. *Journal of Cognitive Neuroscience, 7*, 1–24.

Pribram, K. H., & McGuiness, D. (1975). Arousal, activation, and effort in the control of attention. *Psychological Review, 82*(2), 116–149.

Prichard, R., Schwab, S., & Tillmann, W. A. (1951). Effects of stress and results of medication in different personalities with Parkinson's disease. *Psychosomatic Medicine, 13*, 106–111.

Prutting, C. A., & Kirchner, D. M. (1987). A clinical appraisal of the pragmatic aspects of language. *Journal of Speech and Hearing Disorders, 52*(2), 105–119.

Rachlin, H. C., & Green, L. (1972). Commitment, choice, and self-control. *Journal of the Experimental Analysis of Behavior, 17*, 15–22.

Radinsky, L. B. (1975). Primate brain evolution. *American Scientist, 63*, 656–663.

Rakic, P. (1995). A small step for the cell, a giant leap for mankind: A hypothesis of neocortical expansion during evolution. *Trends in Neurosciences, 18*(9), 383–388.

Ramnani, N., & Owen, A. M. (2004). Anterior prefrontal cortex: Insights into function from anatomy and neuroimaging. *Nature Reviews. Neuroscience, 5*, 184–194.

Rangel, A., Camerer, C., & Montague, P. (2008). A framework for studying the neurobiology of value-based decision making. *Nature Reviews. Neuroscience, 9*, 545–556.

Ray, N., & Strafella, A. P. (2010). Dopamine, reward, and frontostriatal circuitry in impulse control disorders in Parkinson's disease: Insights from functional imaging. *Clinical Electroencephalography and Neuroscience, 41*(2), 87–93.

Razmy, A., Lang, A. E., & Shapiro, C. M. (2004). Predictors of impaired daytime sleep and wakefulness in patients with Parkinson disease treated with older (ergot) vs newer (nonergot) dopamine agonists. *Archives of Neurology, 61*(1), 97–102.

Rescorla, R. A., & Wagner, A. R. (1972). A theory of Pavlovian conditioning: Variations in the effectiveness of reinforcement and nonreinforcement. In A. H. Black & W. F. Prokasy (Eds.), *Classical Conditioning II* (pp. 64–99). New York: Appleton-Century-Crofts.

Ricketts, M., Hammer, R., Manowitz, P., Feng, F., Sage, J., Di Paola, R., et al. (1998). Association of long variants of the dopamine D4 receptor exon 3 repeat polymorphism with Parkinson's disease. *Clinical Genetics, 54*, 33–38.

Riekkinen, M., Kejonen, K., Jakala, P., Soininen, H., & Riekkinen, P., Jr. (1998). Reduction of noradrenaline impairs attention and dopamine depletion slows responses in Parkinson's disease. *European Journal of Neuroscience, 10*, 1429–1435.

Rilling, J. K., & Insel, T. R. (1999). The primate neocortex in comparative perspective using magnetic resonance imaging. *Journal of Human Evolution, 37*, 191–223.

Ringo, J. L. (1991). Neuronal interconnection as a function of brain size. *Brain, Behavior and Evolution, 38*, 1–6.

Rinne, J. O., Portin, R., Ruottinen, H., Nurmi, E., Bergman, J., Haaparanta, M., et al. (2000). Cognitive impairment and the brain dopaminergic system in Parkinson disease: [18F]fluorodopa positron emission tomographic study. *Archives of Neurology, 57*, 470–475.

Rissling, I., Geller, F., Bandmann, O., Stiasny-Kolster, K., Körner, Y., Meindorfner, C., et al. (2004). Dopamine receptor gene polymorphisms in Parkinson's disease patients reporting "sleep attacks.". *Movement Disorders, 19*(11), 1279–1284.

Robert, P. H., Clairet, S., Benoit, M., Koutaich, J., Bertogliatic, C., Tible, O., et al. (2002). The Apathy Inventory: Assessment of apathy and awareness in Alzheimer's disease, Parkinson's disease and mild cognitive impairment. *International Journal of Geriatric Psychiatry, 17*, 1099–1105.

Roese, N. J. (1997). Counterfactual thinking. *Psychological Bulletin, 121*(1), 133–148.

Roese, N. J. (1999). Counterfactual thinking and decision making. *Psychonomic Bulletin & Review*, *6*, 570–578.

Roese, N. J., Hur, T., & Pennington, G. L. (1999). Counterfactual thinking and regulatory focus: Implications for action versus inaction and sufficiency versus necessity. *Journal of Personality and Social Psychology*, *77*(6), 1109–1120.

Ross, D., & Sharp, C. Vuchinich, R., & Spurrett, D. (2003). *Midbrain mutiny: The picoeconomics and neuroeconomics of disordered gambling: Economic theory and cognitive science*. Cambridge, MA: The MIT Press.

Saltzman, J., Strauss, E., Hunter, M., & Archibald, S. (2000). Theory of mind and executive functions in normal human aging and Parkinson's disease. *Journal of the International Neuropsychological Society*, *6*, 781–788.

Sammer, G., Reuter, I., Hullmann, K., Kaps, M., & Vaitl, D. (2006). Training of executive functions in Parkinson's disease. *Journal of the Neurological Sciences*, *248*(1–2), 115–119.

Sandberg, S. G., & Phillips, P. E. M. (2009). Phasic dopaminergic signaling: Implications for Parkinson's disease. In K. Y. Tseng (Ed.), *Cortico-subcortical dynamics in Parkinson's Disease* (pp. 37–54). Totowa, NJ: Humana Press.

Sanides, F. (1964). Structure and function of the human frontal lobe. *Neuropsychologia*, *2*, 209–219.

Sanides, F. (1970). Functional architecture of motor and sensory cortices in primates in the light of a new concept of neocortex evolution. In C. R. Noback & W. Montagna (Eds.), *The primate brain: Advances in primatology* (pp. 137–208). New York: Appleton-Century-Crofts.

Sanides, F. (1972). Representation in the cerebral cortex and its areal lamination patterns. In G. F. Bourne (Ed.), *Structure and function of nervous tissue* (Vol. 5, pp. 329–453). New York: Academic Press.

Santamaria, J., Tolosa, E., & Valles, A. (1986). Parkinson's disease with depression: A possible subgroup of idiopathic parkinsonism. *Neurology*, *36*, 1130–1133.

Savica, R., Rocca, W. A., & Ahlskog, J. E. (2010). When does Parkinson disease start? *Archives of Neurology*, *67*(7), 798–801.

Saxe, R., & Baron-Cohen, S. (2006). The neuroscience of theory of mind. *Social Neuroscience*, *1*(3), 1–9.

Scatton, B., Javoy-Agid, F., Rouquier, L., Dubois, B., & Agid, Y. (1983). Reduction of cortical dopamine, neuroadrenaline, seratonin, and their metabolites in Parkinson's disease. *Brain Research*, *275*, 321–328.

Schenck, C. H., & Mahowald, M. W. (2002). REM sleep behavior disorder: Clinical, developmental, and neuroscience perspectives 16 years after its formal identification. *Sleep*, *25*, 120–130.

Schenck, C. H., Bundlie, S. R., & Mahowald, M. W. (1996). Delayed emergence of a parkinsonian disorder in 38% of 29 older men initially diagnosed with idiopathic rapid eye movement sleep behaviour disorder. *Neurology*, *46*(2), 388–393.

Schenker, N. M., Desgouttes, A. M., & Semendeferi, K. (2005). Neural connectivity and cortical substrates of cognition in hominoids. *Journal of Human Evolution*, *49*(5), 547–569.

Schneider, D., & Sharp, L. (1969). *The dream life of a primitive people*. Ann Arbor, MI: University Microfilms.

Schoenemann, P. T., Sheehan, M. J., & Glotzer, L. D. (2005). Prefrontal white matter volume is disproportionately larger in humans than in other primates. *Nature Neuroscience*, *8*, 242–252.

Schonbar, R. A. (1961). Temporal and emotional factors in the selective recall of dreams. *Journal of Consulting Psychology*, *25*, 67–73.

Schultz, W. (1998). Predictive reward signal of dopamine neurons. *Journal of Neurophysiology*, *80*, 1–27.

Schultz, W., Dayan, P., & Montague, P. R. (1997). A neural substrate of predication and reward. *Science*, *275*, 1593–1599.

Searle, J. R. (1969). *Speech acts*. Cambridge, UK: Cambridge University Press.

Searle, J. R., & Vanderveken, D. (1985). *Foundations of illocutionary logic*. Cambridge, UK: Cambridge University Press.

Sedikides, C., & Spencer, S. (Eds.). (2007). *The self*. New York: Psychology Press, Taylor and Francis Group.

Semendeferi, K., Damasio, H., Frank, R., & Van Hoesen, G. W. (1997). The evolution of the frontal lobes: A volumetric analysis based on three-dimensional reconstructions of magnetic resonance scans of human and ape brains. *Journal of Human Evolution, 32*(4), 375–388.

Semendeferi, K., Lu, A., Schenker, N., & Damasio, H. (2002). Humans and great apes share a large frontal cortex. *Nature Neuroscience, 5*(3), 272–276.

Sesack, S. R., & Grace, A. A. (2010). Cortico-basal ganglia reward network: Microcircuitry. *Neuropsychopharmacology, 35*(1), 27–47.

Shallice, T. (1982). Specific impairments of planning. *Philosophical Transactions of the Royal Society B, Biological Sciences, 298*(1089), 199–209.

Shapiro, K. A., Mottaghy, F. M., Schiller, N. O., Poeppel, T. D., Flub, M. O., & Muller, H. W. (2005). Dissociating neural correlates for nouns and verbs. *NeuroImage, 24*, 1058–1067.

Sheline, Y. I., Barch, D. M., Donnelly, J. M., Olliger, J. M., Snyder, A. Z., Mintun, M. A., et al. (2001). Increased amygdala response to masked emotional faces in depressed subjects resolves with antidepressant treatment: An fMRI study. *Biological Psychiatry, 50*, 651–658.

Shimada, H., Hirano, S., Shinotoh, H., Aotsuka, A., Sato, K., Tanaka, N., et al. (2009). Mapping of brain acetylcholinesterase alterations in Lewy body disease by PET. *Neurology, 73*, 273–278.

Silver, H., Goodman, C., Knoll, G., & Isakov, V. (2004). Brief emotion training improves recognition of facial emotions in chronic schizophrenia. A pilot study. *Psychiatry Research, 128*(2), 174–184.

Silverstein, M. (1976). Hierarchy of features and ergativity. In R. M. W. Dixon (Ed.), *Grammatical categories in Australian languages* (pp. 112–171). Canberra, Australia: Australian Institute of Aboriginal Studies.

Simmons, D. A., Brooks, B. M., & Neill, D. B. (2007). GABAergic inactivation of basolateral amygdala alters behavioral processes other than primary reward of ventral tegmental self-stimulation. *Behavioural Brain Research, 181*(1), 110–117.

Sinforiani, E., Banchieri, L., Zucchella, C., Pacchetti, C., & Sandrini, G. (2004). Cognitive rehabilitation in Parkinson's disease. *Archives of Gerontology and Geriatrics. Supplement, 9*, 387–391.

Sloman, S. A. (1996). The empirical case for two systems of reasoning. *Psychological Bulletin, 119*, 3–22.

Smith, C. (1995). Sleep states and memory processes. *Behavioural Brain Research, 69*(1–2), 137–145.

Smith, K. A., Morris, J. S., Friston, K. J., Cowen, P. J., & Dolan, R. J. (1999). Brain mechanisms associated with depressive relapse and associated cognitive impairment following acute tryptophan depletion. *British Journal of Psychiatry, 174*, 525–529.

Smith, M. T., Perlis, M. L., Chengazi, V. U., Pennington, J., Soeffing, J., Ryan, J. M., et al. (2002). Neuroimaging of NREM sleep in primary insomnia: A Tc-99-HMPAO single photon emission computed tomography study. *Sleep, 25*, 325–335.

Snider, S. R., Fahn, S., Isgreen, W. P., & Cote, L. J. (1976). Primary sensory symptoms in parkinsonism. *Neurology, 26*, 423–429.

Sockeel, P., Dujardin, K., Devos, D., Denève, C., Destée, A., & Defebvre, L. (2006). The Lille apathy rating scale (LARS), a new instrument for detecting and quantifying apathy: Validation in Parkinson's disease. *Journal of Neurology, Neurosurgery, and Psychiatry, 77*, 579–584.

Sprengelmeyer, R., Young, A. W., Mahn, K., Schroeder, U., Woitalla, D., Buttner, T., et al. (2003). Facial expression recognition in people with medicated and unmedicated Parkinson's disease. *Neuropsychologia, 41*, 1047–1057.

Stacy, M. (2002). Sleep disorders in Parkinson's disease: Epidemiology and management. *Drugs & Aging*, *19*(10), 733–739.

Stanley, M., Träskman-Bendz, L., & Dorovini-Zis, K. (1985). Correlations between aminergic metabolites simultaneously obtained from human CSF and brain. *Life Sciences*, *37*, 1279–1286.

Starkstein, S. E., Mayberg, H. S., Leiguarda, R., Preziosi, T. J., & Robinson, R. G. (1992). A prospective longitudinal study of depression, cognitive decline, and physical impairments in patients with Parkinson's disease. *Journal of Neurology, Neurosurgery, and Psychiatry*, *55*(5), 377–382.

Starkstein, S. E., Mayberg, H. S., Preziosi, T. J., Andrezejewski, P., Leiguarda, R., & Robinson, R. G. (1992). Reliability, validity, and clinical correlates of apathy in Parkinson's Disease. *Journal of Neuropsychiatry*, *4*(2), 134–139.

Starkstein, S. E., Merello, M., Jorge, R., Brockman, S., Bruce, D., & Power, B. (2009). The syndromal validity and nosological position of apathy in Parkinson's disease. *Movement Disorders*, *24*(8), 1211–1216.

Starkstein, S. E., Preziosi, T. J., & Robinson, R. G. (1991). Sleep disorders, pain, and depression in Parkinson's disease. *European Neurology*, *31*(6), 352–355.

Stavitsky, K., McNamara, P., Durso, R., Harris, E., Auerbach, S., & Cronin-Golomb, A. (2008). Hallucinations, dreaming and frequent dozing in Parkinson's disease: Impact of right-hemisphere neural networks. *Cognitive and Behavioral Neurology*, *21*(3), 143–149.

Stepansky, R., Holzinger, B., Schmeiser-Rieder, A., Saletu, B., Kunze, M., & Zeitlhofer, J. (1998). Austrian dream behavior: Results of a representative population survey. *Dreaming*, *8*, 23–30.

Stephan, H., & Andy, O. J. (1969). Quantitative comparative neuroanatomy of primates: An attempt at a phylogenetic interpretation. *Annals of the New York Academy of Sciences*, *167*, 370–387.

Stern, Y., Mayeux, R., & Cote, L. (1984). Reaction time and vigilance in Parkinson's disease. Possible role of altered norepinephrine metabolism. *Archives of Neurology*, *41*, 1086–1089.

Stern, Y., Tang, M. X., Jacobs, D. M., Sano, M., Marder, K., Bell, K., et al. (1998). Prospective comparative study of the evolution of probable Alzheimer's disease and Parkinson's disease dementia. *International Neuropsychological Society*, *4*(3), 279–284.

Stickgold, R. (1998). Sleep: Off-line memory reprocessing. *Trends in Cognitive Sciences*, *2*, 484–492.

Stickgold, R., Hobson, J. A., Fosse, R., & Fosse, M. (2001). Sleep, learning, and dreams: Off-line memory reprocessing. *Science*, *294*(5544), 1052–1057.

Strack, F., & Deutsch, R. (2004). Reflective and impulsive determinants of social behavior. *Personality and Social Psychology Review*, *8*, 220–247.

Strauch, I., & Meier, B. (1996). *In search of dreams: Results of experimental dream research*. Albany, NY: State University of New York Press.

Stroop, J. R. (1935). Studies of interference in serial verbal reactions. *Journal of Experimental Psychology*, *18*, 643–662.

Suri, R. E. (2002). TD models of reward predictive responses in dopamine neurons. *Neural Networks*, *15*(4), 523–533.

Sutton, R. S., & Barto, A. G. (1990). Time-derivative models of Pavlovian reinforcement. In M. Gabriel & J. Moore (Eds.), *Learning and computational neuroscience: Foundations of adaptive networks* (pp. 497–537). Cambridge, MA: The MIT Press.

Sutton, R. S., & Barto, A. G. (1998). *Reinforcement learning: An introduction*. Cambridge, MA: The MIT Press.

Symons, C. S., & Johnson, B. T. (1997). The self-reference effect in memory: A meta-analysis. *Psychological Bulletin*, *121*(3), 371–394.

Synofzik, M., Vosgerau, G., & Newen, A. (2008). Beyond the comparator model: A multifactorial two-step account of agency. *Consciousness and Cognition*, *17*(1), 219–239.

Takahata, R., & Moghaddam, B. (1998). Glutamatergic regulation of basal and stimulus-activated dopamine release in the prefrontal cortex. *Journal of Neurochemistry, 71*, 1443–1450.

Taylor, A. E., & Saint-Cyr, J. A. (1992). Executive function. In J. L. Cummings & S. J. Huber (Eds.), *Parkinson's disease: Behavioural and neuropsychological aspects* (pp. 74–85). New York: Oxford University Press.

Taylor, A. E., & Saint-Cyr, J. A. (1995). The neuropsychology of Parkinson's disease. *Brain and Cognition, 28*(3), 281–296.

Taylor, A. E., Saint-Cyr, J. A., & Lang, A. E. (1986). Frontal lobe dysfunction in Parkinson's disease. The cortical focus of neostriatal outflow. *Brain, 109*(5), 845–883.

Tedlock, B. (1992). *Dreaming: Anthropological and psychological interpretations.* Santa Fe, NM: School of America Research Press.

Terzi, A., Papapetropoulos, S., & Kouvelas, E. D. (2005). Past tense formation and comprehension of passive sentences in Parkinson's disease: Evidence from Greek. *Brain and Language, 94*(3), 297–303.

Thiel, A., Hilker, R., Kessler, J., Habedank, B., Herholz, K., & Heiss, W. D. (2003). Activation of basal ganglia loops in idiopathic Parkinson's disease: A PET study. *Journal of Neural Transmission, 110*, 1289–1301.

Tomer, R., & Aharon-Peretz, J. (2004). Novelty seeking and harm avoidance in Parkinson's disease: Effects of asymmetric dopamine deficiency. *Journal of Neurology, Neurosurgery, and Psychiatry, 75*(7), 972–975.

Tomer, R., Levin, B. E., & Weiner, W. J. (1993). Side of onset of motor symptoms influences cognition in Parkinson's disease. *Annals of Neurology, 34*(4), 579–584.

Torack, R. M., & Morris, J. C. (1988). The association of ventral tegmental area histopathology with adult dementia. *Archives of Neurology, 45*(5), 497–501.

Troster, A. I., & Woods, S. P. (2003). Neuropsychological aspects of Parkinson's disease and parkinsonian syndromes. In R. Pahwa, K. E. Lyons, & W. C. Koller (Eds.), *Handbook of Parkinson's disease* (pp. 127–157). New York: Dekker.

Tse, W. S., & Bond, A. J. (2005). The application of the Temperament and Character Inventory (TCI) in predicting general social adaptation and specific social behaviors in a dyadic interaction. *Journal of Applied Social Psychology, 35*(8), 1571–1586.

Tsuno, N., Besset, A., & Ritchie, K. (2005). Sleep and depression. *Journal of Clinical Psychiatry, 66*, 1254–1269.

Turner, R. S. (2002). Idiopathic rapid eye movement sleep behavior disorder is a harbinger of dementia with Lewy bodies. *Journal of Geriatric Psychiatry and Neurology, 15*(4), 195–199.

Tversky, A., & Kahneman, D. (1981). The framing of decisions and the psychology of choice. *Science, 211*(4481), 453–458.

Uddin, L. Q., Iacoboni, M., & Lange, C. (2007). The self and social cognition: The role of cortical midline structures and mirror neurons. *Trends in Cognitive Sciences, 11*(4), 153–157.

Uitti, R. J., Baba, Y., Whaley, N. R., Wszolek, Z. K., & Putzke, J. D. (2005). Parkinson disease: Handedness predicts asymmetry. *Neurology, 64*, 1925–1930.

Uylings, H. B. M., & van Eden, C. G. (1990). Qualitative and quantitative comparison of the prefrontal cortex in rat and in primates, including humans. In H. B. M. Uylings, C. G. Van Eden, J. P. C. De Bruin, M. A. Corner, & M. G. P. Feenstra (Eds.), *Progress in brain research* (Vol. 85, pp. 31–62). Amsterdam, The Netherlands: Elsevier.

Van Moffaert, M. M. M. P. (1994). Sleep disorders and depression: The 'chicken and egg' situation. *Journal of Psychosomatic Research, 38*(Suppl. 1), 9–13.

Vann, B., & Alperstein, N. (2000). Dream sharing as social interaction. *Dreaming, 10*, 111–120.

van Reekum, R., Stuss, D. T., & Ostrander, L. (2005). Apathy: Why care. *Journal of Neuropsychiatry and Clinical Neurosciences, 17,* 7–19.

Van Tol, H., Bunzow, J. R., Guan, H. C., Sunahara, R. K., Seeman, P., Niznik, H. B., et al. (1991). Cloning of the gene for a human dopamine D4 receptor with high affinity for the antipsychotic clozapine. *Nature, 350,* 610–614.

Vogel, G. W., Thurmond, A., Gibbons, P., Sloan, K., & Walker, M. (1975). REM sleep reduction effects on depression syndromes. *Archives of General Psychiatry, 32,* 765–777.

Vogeley, K., May, M., Ritzl, A., Falkai, P., Zilles, K., & Fink, G. R. (2004). Neural correlates of first-person perspective as one constituent of human selfconsciousness. *Journal of Cognitive Neuroscience, 16*(5), 817–827.

Volk, S. A., Kaendler, S. H., Hertel, A., Maul, F. D., Manoocheri, R., Weber, R., et al. (1997). Can response to partial sleep deprivation in depressed patients be predicted by regional changes of cerebral blood flow? *Psychiatry Research: Neuroimaging, 75*(2), 67–74.

Volk, S. A., Kaendler, S. H., Weber, R., Georgi, K., Maul, R. Hertel, A., et al. (1992). Evaluation of the effect of total sleep deprivation on cerebral blood flow using single photon emission computerized tomography. *Acta Neurologica Scandinavica, 86,* 473–483.

Volpato, C., Signorini, M., Meneghello, F., & Semenza, C. (2009). Cognitive and personality features in Parkinson Disease: 2 sides of the same coin? *Cognitive and Behavioral Neurology, 22*(4), 258–263.

Voon, V., Hassan, K., Zurowski, M., de Souza, M., Thomsen, T., Fox, S., et al. (2006). Prevalence of repetitive and reward-seeking behaviors in Parkinson's disease. *Neurology, 67,* 1254–1257.

Voon, V., Thomsen, T., Miyasaki, J. M., de Souza, M., Shafro, A., Fox, S. H., et al. (2007). Factors associated with dopaminergic drug-related pathological gambling in Parkinson disease. *Archives of Neurology, 64*(2), 212–216.

Voorn, P., Vanderschuren, L. J., Groenewegen, H. J., Robbins, T. W., & Pennartz, C. M. (2004). Putting a spin on the dorsal-ventral divide of the striatum. *Trends in Neurosciences, 27,* 468–474.

Waelti, P., Dickinson, A., & Schultz, W. (2001). Dopamine responses comply with basic assumptions of formal learning theory. *Nature, 412,* 43–48.

Waite, L. M., Broe, G. A., Grayson, D. A., & Creasey, H. (2001). Preclinical syndromes predict dementia: The Sydney older persons study. *Journal of Neurology, Neurosurgery, and Psychiatry, 71*(3), 296–302.

Walker, M. P., Brakefield, T., Hobson, J. A., & Stickgold, R. (2003). Sleep and the time course of motor skill learning. *Learning & Memory (Cold Spring Harbor, N.Y.), 10*(4), 275–284.

Wan, D. C., Law, L. K., Ip, D. T., Cheung, W. T., Ho, W. K., Tsim, K. W., et al. (1999). Lack of allelic association of dopamine D4 receptor gene polymorphisms with Parkinson's disease in a Chinese population. *Movement Disorders, 14*(2), 225–229.

Ward, C. D., Duvoisin, R. C., Ince, S. E., Nutt, J. D., Putnam, J. J., et al. (1984). Parkinson's disease in twins. In R. G. Hassler & F. Christ (Eds.), *Advances in neurology* (Vol. 40, pp. 341–344). New York: Raven Press.

Weaver, F. M., Follett, K., Stern, M., Hur, K., Harris, C., Marks, W. J., Jr., et al. (2009). Bilateral deep brain stimulation vs best medical therapy for patients with advanced Parkinson disease: a randomized controlled trial. *Journal of the American Medical Association, 301*(1), 63–73.

Wegelin, J., McNamara, P., Durso, R., Brown, A., & McLaren, D. (2005). Correlates of excessive daytime sleepiness in Parkinson's disease. *Parkinsonism & Related Disorders, 11*(7), 441–448.

Wegner, D. M. (2003). The mind's best trick: How we experience conscious will. *Trends in Cognitive Sciences, 7*(2), 65–69.

Weinberger, D. R., Berman, K. F., & Illowsky, B. P. (1988). Physiological dysfunction of dorsolateral prefrontal cortex in schizophrenia III: A new cohort and evidence for monoaminergic mechanism. *Archives of General Psychiatry, 45,* 609–615.

Weinberger, D. R., Berman, K. K., & Zec, R. F. (1986). Physiologic dysfunction of dorsolateral prefrontal cortex in schizophrenia: Regional blood flow evidence. *Archives of General Psychiatry, 43,* 114–124.

Weintraub, D., Siderowf, A. D., Potenza, M. N., Goveas, J., Morales, K. H., Duda, J. E., et al. (2006). Association of dopamine agonist use with impulse control disorders in Parkinson disease. *Archives of Neurology, 63,* 969–973.

Wester, P., Bergstrom, U., Eriksson, A., Gezellius, C., Hardy, J., & Winblad, B. (1990). Ventricular cerebrospinal fluid monoamine transmitter and metabolite concentrations reflect human brain neurochemistry in autopsy cases. *Journal of Neurochemistry, 54,* 1148–1156.

Wetter, T. C., Brunner, H., Hogl, B., Yassouridis, A., Trenkwalder, C., & Friess, E. (2001). Increased alpha activity in REM sleep in de novo patients with Parkinson's disease. *Movement Disorders, 16,* 928–933.

Wheeler, M. A., Stuss, D. T., & Tulving, E. (1997). Toward a theory of episodic memory: The frontal lobes and autonoetic consciousness. *Psychological Bulletin, 121,* 331–354.

Whitehouse, P. J., Hedreen, J. C., White, C. L., III, & Price, D. L. (1983). Basal forebrain neurons in the dementia of Parkinson disease. *Annals of Neurology, 13,* 243–248.

Whiting, E., Copland, D., & Angwin, A. (2005). Verb and context processing in Parkinson's disease. *Journal of Neurolinguistics, 18*(3), 259–276.

Williams, G. V., & Goldman-Rakic, P. S. (1995). Modulation of memory fields by dopamine D1 receptors in prefrontal cortex. *Nature, 376,* 572–575.

Wilson, M. A., & McNaughton, B. L. (1994). Reactivation of hippocampal ensemble memories during sleep. *Science, 265,* 676–679.

Winokur, A., Gary, K. A., Rodner, S., Rae-Red, C., Fernando, A. T., & Szuba, M. P. (2001). Depression, sleep physiology, and antidepressant drugs. *Depression and Anxiety, 14*(1), 19–28.

Wolfe, F., Smythe, H., Yunus, M., Bennett, R., Bombardier, C., & Goldenberg, D. (1990). The American College of Rheumatology 1990 criteria for the classification of fibromyalgia. Report of the Multicenter Criteria Committee. *Arthritis and Rheumatism, 33,* 160–172.

Wolters, E., & Scheltens, P. (Eds.). (1995). *Mental dysfunction in Parkinson's disease.* Dordrecht, The Netherlands: ICG.

Wolters, E. Ch., van der Werf, Y. D., & van den Heuvel, O. A. (2008). Parkinson's disease-related disorders in the impulsive-compulsive spectrum. *Journal of Neurology, 255,* 48–56.

Woods, S. P., & Troster, A. I. (2003). Prodromal frontal/executive dysfunction predicts incident dementia in Parkinson's disease. *Journal of the International Neuropsychological Society, 9*(1), 17–24.

Wu, J. C., Buchsbaum, M., & Bunney, W. E. (2001). Clinical neurochemical implications of sleep deprivation's effects on the anterior cingulate of depressed responders. *Neuropharmacology, 25,* S74–S78.

Wu, J. C., Buchsbaum, M. S., Gillin, J. C., Tang, C., Cadwell, S., Wiegand, M., et al. (1999). Prediction of antidepressant effects of sleep deprivation by metabolic rates in the ventral anterior cingulate and medial prefrontal cortex. *American Journal of Psychiatry, 156,* 1149–1158.

Wu, J. C., Gillin, G. C., Buchsbaum, M. S., Hershey, R., & Johnson, J. C. (1992). Effects of sleep deprivation on brain metabolism of depressed patients. *American Journal of Psychiatry, 149,* 538–543.

Wu, J. C., Gillin, J. C., Buchsbaum, M. S., Schachat, C., Darnall, L. A., Keator, D. B., et al. (2008). Sleep deprivation PET correlations of Hamilton symptom improvement ratings with changes in relative glucose metabolism in patients with depression. *Journal of Affective Disorders, 107,* 181–186.

Yip, J. T., Lee, T. M., Ho, S. L., Tsang, K. L., & Li, L. S. (2003). Emotion recognition in patients with idiopathic Parkinson's disease. *Movement Disorders, 18*(10), 1115–1122.

Ylvisaker, M., McPherson, K., Kayes, N., & Pellett, E. (2008). Metaphoric identity mapping: Facilitating goal setting and engagement in rehabilitation after traumatic brain injury. *Neuropsychological Rehabilitation, 18*(5–6), 713–741.

Yoshimura, N., & Kawamura, M. (2005). Impairment of social cognition in Parkinson's disease. *Brain and Nerve*, *57*(2), 107–113.

Zhang, K., & Sejnowski, T. J. (2000). A universal scaling law between gray matter and white matter of cerebral cortex. *Proceedings of the National Academy of Sciences of the United States of America*, *97*, 5621–5626.

Zilles, K., Armstrong, E., Moser, K. H., Schleicher, A., & Stephan, H. (1989). Gyrification in the cerebral cortex of primates. *Brain, Behavior and Evolution*, *34*, 143–150.

Zilles, K., Armstrong, E., Schleicher, A., & Kretschmann, H. J. (1988). The human pattern of gyrification in the cerebral cortex. *Anatomy and Embryology*, *179*, 173–179.

Index

Agency
  feeling of, 42, 82–83
  judgment of, 42
Agentic personality styles, dopamine and, 74–75
Agentic self, 41–42, 54–56. *See also under*
    Minimal self
  cognitive operations of, 57–60, 58f, 68, 74
    step 1: identifying values to be striven for,
      60–61, 77
    step 2: prioritizing values into long-term goals,
      61–62, 77–78
    step 3: deciding which goals to pursue, 62–65,
      78–81
    step 4: developing plans to attain goals, 65–66, 82
    step 5: initiating goal pursuit, 66–67, 82–84
    step 6: monitoring and adjusting, 67
  defined, 37
  deflationary accounts of, 72–74
  evolution of prefrontal networks subserving,
    114–115
  functions of, 105
  models of, 47, 47f, 48, 120
  neuropsychiatric disorders as impairments of
    subcomponents of, 69–72
  personality traits associated with, 111
    evolution of, 111–112
  properties of, 42–50
  prospect theory and, 53–54
  regret theory and, 53
  rehabilitation of (*see* Rehabilitation)
Agentic self system, 73, 76, 86–88, 102, 109, 114,
    171, 177
  language deficits, speech act processing, and,
    129, 132–136
  mood disorder as dysfunction in, 155, 170
  right prefrontal cortex and, 133
  sleep disorders and, 137–138

Aggression, 90
  REM sleep-related dreams simulate, 147–148
Akinesia. *See* Freezing
Albert, M., 91
Alzheimer's disease (AD), 76
Alzheimer's disease dementia (ADD), 172
Amygdala, 155–156
Anarchic hand, 46
Anger, 159–160
Animacy hierarchy, 135–136, 135f
Anxiety, 88–89, 143–144, 144f, 161–162
Anxiety disorders, 90
Apathy, 166–168
  clinical phenomenology, 168
  dementia and, 173
  diagnostic criteria, 167, 167t
  Levy-Dubois subtypes, 168–169
  measurement, 169
"Apathy plus" syndromes, 168
Apomorphine, 183
Asymmetry in PD, 19, 23
Au, R., 91
Autonomic nervous system (ANS) dysfunction,
    185
Autonomic nervous system (ANS) function, 19

Bandura, A., 37, 42, 45
Barbas, H., 119
Barto, A. G., 28–29
Basolateral nucleus, 156
Bechara, A., 58–59
Ben-Yishay, Y., 187
Bodily awareness, 38–41
Bodily self, 40, 41, 136. *See also* Minimal self
Booth, G., 90
Bower, J. H., 88–89
Braak, H., 21–22, 22t

Bradykinesia, 17
Brain dysfunction in PD, 75–77. *See also specific topics*
Brain evolution, 114–115
Brain injury, 187–189
Brain stimulation, deep, 4–5
Branching control, 64
Brodmann area 10 (BA10), 62–64
Brown, A., 78, 79t, 91, 141, 147, 192
Burns, K., 58–59

Calne, S., 143–144
Camerer, C., 59–62
Cappaert, K., 123, 125
Carbidopa, 4, 5
Cascade model (PFC function), 64, 65t
Catech-*O*-methyltransferase (COMT), 6
Caudate, 27
Cause-effect folk psychology, 45–46
Cerebrospinal fluid homovanillic acid (CSF HVA), 32
Charcot, Jean-Martin, 3
Cholinergic contributions to dementia, 175–176
Clare, L., 188
Clark, J., 33, 133
Claustrophobia, 90
Cloute, K., 188–189
Commissives (speech acts), 124
Comparator model of agentic self, 47, 47f, 48
Comprehension, 191–192. *See also* Speech act production and comprehension
sentence, 133–134
Compulsive eating, 185
Compulsive gambling, 184
Compulsive spending, 185
Conformism, social, 91
Conscientiousness, 91
Control. *See* Agentic self
Correlated evolution (brain), 114–115
Counterfactual comparisons, 51–53
Counterfactual Inference Test (CIT), 79, 79t
Counterfactual processing, 29, 51, 78–80
Counterfactuals
acceptable, 52
defined, 78
Cytoarchitectonic theory, evolutionary, 119–121

Damasio, A. R., 58–59
Damasio, H., 58–59
Darlington, R. B., 115
Decision accuracy, lexical, 128, 128t
Decision making, 49
models of, 50

Decision-making capacities of agentic self, 59–60, 62–65, 78–81
Decisions under risk *vs.* uncertainty, 49–50
Declarations (speech acts), 124
Deep brain stimulation (DBS), 4–5
Default network of brain sites, 67
Deflationary accounts of the self, 72–74
Delusions, 176
Dementia, 171
clinical phenomenology and pathophysiology, 172–179
PD patients with *vs.* without, 76–77
Dementia with Lewy bodies (DLB), 172
Denial, 158–159
Dependent personality, 90
Depression, 162
brain mechanisms of, 149–152
cognitive deficit and, 165
neurochemical contributions to, 163–164
prefrontal-limbic loops in, 164
REM sleep indices enhanced in, 150–151
treatments for, 166
Depressive symptomatology, 162–163
Depressiveness, 88–89
Desgouttes, A. M., 117
Developmental constraints model of brain evolution, 115
Directives (speech acts), 124
Dopamine (DA)
and executive cognitive functions, 31–33
models of, and PD neuropsychiatry, 35–36
Dopamine (DA) agonists, 153, 182
Dopamine dysregulation syndrome (DDS), 183, 186
Dopamine-four-receptor (DRD4) variants, 113–114
Dopamine (DA) receptors, families of, 27
Dopamine (DA) release, tonic *vs.* phasic mechanisms of, 27–28
Dopamine (DA) signaling
interaction of phasic and tonic, 33–34
prediction-error theory of, 30–31
role of temporal discounting in, 30–31, 83
Dopaminergic anatomy and physiology, 25–27
Dopaminergic contributions to dementia, 173–174
Dopaminergic pathways of brain, 25–26, 26f
Dorsal prefrontal cortex (dPFC), 87, 150–152
Dorsolateral prefrontal cortex (DLPFC), 64–66, 75–77, 155, 170
Dorsolateral prefrontal cortex (DLPFC)-striatal loop, 81

Dorsolateral prefrontal cortex (DLPFC) sites, hypoactivation of, 150
Dreaming, importance of vivid, 147
Dreams, vivid
predicting later onset of PD, 148
Drug-induced psychosis, 176
Dubois, B., 168–169
Durso, R., 19, 31, 33, 34, 77–78, 79t, 91, 101, 102, 103f, 105, 107, 108t, 123, 125, 132, 133, 141, 176, 189, 192
Durstewitz, D., 34
Dyskinesias, 5, 7. See also Motor symptoms

Efference copy, 48
Ego-identity change, 187–188
Emotional processing, 157–160. See also Social emotional perception/expression
deficits in, 160–161
of particularized implicatures, 129–131, 130t
Empathy, 104. See also Mentalizing abilities
Enactment behaviors, nighttime dream-related, 148
Environmental toxins, 20
Error correction, 46–47
Euteneuer, F., 81
Evolutionary cytoarchitectonic theory, 119–121
Evolutionary history of prefrontal cortex in mammals, 115–116
Excessive daytime sleepiness (EDS), 143–144
Executive cognitive functions (ECFs), 25, 75
deficits/impairment in, 83–84, 112
diminution of phasic signaling and, 31–33
personality traits and, 102
Executive control system, 63, 85, 137, 160, 181–182. See also Agentic self
Expected utility (EU) theory, 61
Expressives (speech acts), 124
Extraversion, 74, 75, 114

Feed-forward comparator models, 67
Finlay, B. L., 115
Fleming, J. A. E., 143–144
Forethought, 43
Forward modeling, 46–48
Fotopoulou, A., 187–188
Fox, Michael J., 10
Free radicals, 20
Freezing, 18
Frontal-basal ganglia loops
Frontal lobe. See Executive cognitive functions
Future directedness, 45

Gallagher, S., 37–38, 40
Gambling, pathologic, 184
Game of Dice Task (GDT), 81
Gene therapies, 5
Genes linked to PD, 20, 21t
Genetics, 20–21, 89
Gilles de la Tourette, Georges. See Tourette, Georges Gilles de la
Glosser, G., 88
Glotzer, L. D., 118
Goals. See under Agentic self: cognitive operations of
Graboys, Thomas, 10–11, 158
Gracey, F., 188
Grammatical processing, 133–134. See also Language structure
Grossman, M., 133

Hallucinations
sleep and, 148–149
visual, 176–177
Harm avoidance (HA), 35, 91–92
Harris, E., 19, 34, 77, 91, 101, 102, 103f, 105, 107, 108t, 123, 189
Hobbes, Thomas, 8, 11
Hoehn-Yahr (HY) Parkinson's Disease Rating Scale, 13, 15t
Holtgraves, T., 123, 125, 126t–128t, 130t, 175
Homovanillic acid (HVA), 32
Hubble, J. P., 88
Hypersexuality, 184

Identity-oriented goal setting (IOG), 189
Illocutionary force (speech), 125
Implementation intentions, 43–44
Implicatures, 124
comprehending particularized, 129–131, 130t
defined, 124
generalized vs. particularized, 124–125
Impulse control disorders (ICDs), 181–182, 186
clinical phenomenology, 184–186
Impulsive valuation and responding, inhibition of, 57
Industriousness, 90
Insomnia, 142–143
Intelligence, 7–8, 90
Intentional binding, 43
Intentionality, 42–43, 74
Intentions, conscious, 46
Interference cost, 84
Interpersonal relationships, 159–160

Introverted premorbid personality type, 88
Intuition *vs.* reasoning, 59
Iowa Gambling Task (IGT), 80–82

John Paul II, Pope, 8–10
Johnson, P., 106

Kahneman, D., 52
Kinesia paradoxica, 17
Koechlin, E., 64–65
Koller, W. C., 88
Kondracke, Milly, 11
Krueger, M., 33, 133

Language deficit, 123–124
Language-related deficits, 69. *See also* Speech
   acts
Language structure. *See also* Grammatical
   processing
   agency and, 134–136
Left-onset PD (LPD), 19
Levodopa (*L*-dopa; LD), 4–7, 161
   and executive cognitive functions, 31–33
   and mood, 166
Levy, R., 168–169
Lexical decision accuracy, 128, 128t
Libet, B., 46
Limbic-orbitofrontal (OF) loop, 81
Limbic-PFC loop, 164, 182
Linguistic Inquiry and Word Count (LIWC)
   program, 133
Locus ceruleus (LC), 174
Long 7 repeats allele (L-DRD4), 112
Lynch, A., 78, 79t, 192

MACH-IV, 107
Machiavellian personality types, 107–108, 108t
Machover, S., 90–91
Major depressive disorder (MDD), 162, 163, 165,
   166
Maneb, 20
Mania, 177
Markus, H., 54–55
Matching laws, 30
Mayberg, H. S., 149–150, 164
McGuiness, D., 120
McLaren, D., 91, 102, 105, 141, 147
McNamara, Patrick, 19, 31, 33, 34, 58f, 77–78, 79t,
   91, 101, 102, 103f, 105–107, 108t, 123, 125,
   126t–128t, 130t, 132, 133, 141, 147, 163, 175, 176,
   189, 192
Memory, autobiographical, 102, 103f, 104
Memory deficits, 85

Mentalizing abilities, 104–107, 109, 189. *See also*
   Theory of mind
Metacognitive strategy instruction (MSI), 193
Metaphoric identity mapping, 189
Miller, D. T., 52
Mind. *See* Theory of mind
Minimal self
   access to current, 104
   action as requiring temporary suppression of,
      38
   agentic self and, 37, 68, 83, 85–86, 119, 123, 164,
      166, 170, 181–182
   bodily self and, 40–41
   components, 40
   control of agentic self over operations of, 74–75
   "default network" and, 38
   Gallagher on, 37–38
   initiating goal pursuit by inhibiting impulses
      associated with, 66–67
   narrative self and, 37, 38
   nature of, 37–38
   neural structures that mediate, 170
   REM sleep and, 137–139
Minnesota Multiphasic Personality Inventory
   (MMPI), 88–89
Mitchell, A., 188–189
Monoamine oxidase (MAO) inhibitors, 6
Montague, P., 59–62
Mood disorder. *See also* Depression
   as dysfunction in agentic self system, 155, 170
Moralism, 90
Mosaic evolution, model of, 114–115
Motor symptoms. *See also* Dyskinesias
   drugs used to treat, 6, 6t, 7
Movement Disorder Society (MDS), 16, 172
MPTP (1-methyl-4-phenyl-1,2,3,
   6-tetrahydropyridine), 13
Mutability, rules of, 52

Narrative self, 37, 38, 41–42
Naylor, E., 188
NEO Personality Inventory, 88
Neocortical evolution, 115
Neuropsychiatric disorders of PD, ix, 12. *See also*
   specific topics
   top-down *vs.* bottom-up approach to, ix–x
Neuroscience of Religious Experience, The
   (McNamara), 58f
Norepinephrine (NE), 32
   and ECF deficit, 174
Novelty seeking (NS), 74–75, 91–92, 114, 120
Nucleus accumbens circuit (NAC), 27, 156
Nurius, P., 54–55

Obler, L. K., 91
Orbitofrontal cortex (OFC), 61, 62
Othello syndrome, 176
Oxidative stress, 20

Pain, 19
Pal, P. K., 143–144
Pandya, D. N., 119
Paraquat, 20
Parkinson, James, 3
Parkinsonian personality. *See* Personality,
  parkinsonian
Parkinson's disease (PD). *See also specific topics*
  case studies, 7–12
  causes, 20–23
  clinical symptoms and course, 16–19
  diagnostic criteria, 13–16, 14t
  epidemiology, 2
  famous people suspected of having, 8–12
  history of the study of, 3–5
  nature of, 1–3
  neuropathology and progression, 21–22
  nonmotor features, 18–19
  overview, 1, 2
  pathologic stages, 21–22, 22t
  risk factors in progression to, 137, 138t
  treatment of
    gold standard therapy for, 5–7
    history of, 3–5
Parkinson's disease dementia (PDD). *See*
  Dementia
Parkinson's disease patients with dementia
  (PDD). *See* Dementia
Parkinson's disease-related spatial covariance
  pattern (PDRP), 76
Pavlovian valuation system, 61
Penn, David, 190
Perception-action cycle, 63
Periodic limb movement disorder, 145
Personality, parkinsonian, 87–89, 108–109
  persists through the course of the illness, 89–91,
    100–102
  research on, 88–101t
Personality styles, agentic
  dopamine and, 74–75
Personality traits
  associated with agentic self, 111
  evolution of, 111–112
  associated with PD, 7–8, 111
Personality types, Machiavellian, 107–108, 108t
Personhood, 39–40
Perspective taking abilities, 41, 104. *See also*
  Mentalizing abilities

Pessimism, 88–89
Pesticides, 20
Phasic signaling. *See also* Dopamine (DA)
  signaling
  ECF deficits and the diminution of, 31–33
Planning, 71–72, 85
Points of view, 53
Possible worlds, modeling of, 48
Posttraumatic stress disorder (PTSD), 141
Postural instability, 18
Pragmatics (component of language), 123
  speech acts and, 124–125
Pramipexole, 183
Prediction-error theory of DA signaling, 30–31
Prefrontal cortex (PFC), 19, 26–27, 31, 36, 62–68,
    75. *See also* Dorsal prefrontal cortex;
    Dorsolateral prefrontal cortex
  agentic self system and, 133
  anxiety and, 161–162
  connectivity differences, 118–119
  evolutionary history, 115–116
  size differences, 116–119
Prefrontal networks subserving agentic self,
  evolution of, 114–115
Prefrontal-subcortical circuits, 178, 178t
Premorbid personality. *See also* Personality
  agentic self and, 69, 137
  evidence for, 87–89
  psychoanalytic conceptualization of, 90, 181–182
Premorbid personality type, 7–8, 87–88
Pribram, K. H., 120
Prichard, R., 90
Prospect theory (PT) and the agentic self, 53–54,
  61
Prospective memory, as guiding action, 48–49
Prospective memory deficits, 85
Psychosis, 176–177
  pathophysiology, 177–179
Punding, 185–186
Putamen, 27

Rage, 159
Rangel, A., 59–62
Reaction formation, 182
Readiness potential, 46
Reasoning *vs.* intuition, 59
Rehabilitation, 187, 193–194
  cognitive, 192–193
  is possible only for a person, not a syndrome,
    187–189
Rehabilitation approaches directed at the self,
  189
Relational self, 40

Relationships, 159–160
REM (rapid eye movement) sleep, 137–138.
    See also Sleep disturbances
    activates ventral system and deactivates dorsal
        system, 150
REM sleep behavior disorder (RBD), 16, 89,
    145–147
    predicting later onset of PD, 148
REM sleep deprivation, 151–152
REM sleep disturbances, special role of, 140–141
REM sleep indices enhanced in depression,
    150–151
REM sleep-related dreams simulate aggression,
    147–148
Repetitive transcranial magnetic stimulation
    (rTMS), 166
Representatives (speech acts), 124
Rescorla, R. A., 29
Restless legs syndrome (RLS), 145
Reward dependence, 91–92
Right-onset PD (RPD), 19
Rigidity, 18, 90

Samii, A., 143–144
Sammer, G., 192
Sanides, F., 119
Schenker, N. M., 117
Schizophrenia, 8
Schoenemann, P. T., 118
Schwab, S., 90
Seamans, J. K., 34
Self, 72. *See also* Agentic self
    altered sense of, 102
    deflationary accounts of the, 72–74
Self-concept, 38, 187–188. *See also* Agentic self
Self-reactiveness, 43–44
Self-reference effect, 66–67
Self-reflectiveness, 44–45
Seltzer, B., 119
Semendeferi, K., 117
Sensory suppression, 48
Sentence processing, 133–134
Sexual disorders, 184–185
Sheehan, M. J., 118
Silverstein, M., 135–136
Sinemet, 5
Sinforiani, E., 192
Situational cues, 44
Sleep, hallucinations and, 148–149
Sleep apnea, 145
"Sleep attacks," 143
Sleep centers, neuropathology of PD and,
    141–142

Sleep disorder breathing, 145
Sleep disturbances, 152–153
    agentic self system and, 137–138
    mental dysfunction and, 139–140
    profile of, 142–148
    as source of neuropsychiatric disorders, 138–139
Sleepiness, excessive daytime, 143–144
Smith, D., 147
Social cognition, 105, 193
Social Cognition Interaction Training (SCIT),
    190–192
Social cognitive processing deficits, 189
    how personality traits contribute to psychiatric
        symptoms via, 102–104
Social conformism, 91
Social emotional perception/expression, 190
Social functions, 105
Social roles/social scripts, 106–107
Speech act processing, 132–134
Speech act production and comprehension, 69,
    124–125, 132
    experimental findings on, 125–132
    grammatical and sentence comprehension,
        133–134
Speech act recognition deficit, 128–129
Speech acts, 123–124
    pragmatics and, 124–125
    types of, 124
Standard Social Skills Rehabilitation Training
    (SSSRT) program, 188
Stavitsky, K., 19
Stickgold, R., 147
Stroop Test, 84
Subthalamic nucleus, stimulation of, 4–5
Suggestibility, 90
Summerfield, C., 64–65
Supplemental motor area (SMA), 26, 27, 46
Sutton, R. S., 28–29
Szent-Imrey, O., 19

Temperament and Character Inventory (TCI),
    101, 107
Temporal difference (TD) algorithm, 28–29
Temporal discounting, 83
    in DA signaling, role of, 30–31, 83
    defined, 49
Theory of mind (ToM), 41, 104–106, 189. *See also*
    Mentalizing abilities
Tillmann, W. A., 90
Tourette, Georges Gilles de la, 3–4
Tower of London (TOL) task, 65–66, 82
Tranel, D., 58–59
Trauma, 141

Traumatic brain injury (TBI), 187–189
Tremor, 17–18
Tri-dimensional Personality Questionnaire
 (TPQ), 91, 101
Twin studies, 89, 96t, 100–101t

UK Parkinson's Disease Society Brain Bank
 diagnostic criteria, 13, 14t
Unified Parkinson's Disease Rating Scale
 (UPDRS), 15–16
Unified self system, complexity of, 39–42

Value-based decision making, 59–60
Values
 prioritizing, 61–62, 77–78
 for which to strive, identifying, 60–61, 77
Ventral striatum, 157
Ventral tegmental area (VTA), 26, 27, 141–142,
 173
Ventromedial PFC, 66
Verbs, processing of, 132–133
Vibration therapy, 3–4
Visceromotor circuit, 165

Wagner, A. R., 29
Wegelin, J., 141
Wegner, D. M., 46
Will power, 58–59
Working memory, 25, 33–34, 104, 174. *See also*
 Executive cognitive functions

Yates, P., 188–189